Clinical Manual for Assessment and Treatment of Suicidal Patients

Clinical Manual for Assessment and Treatment of Suicidal Patients

John A. Chiles, M.D.

Clinical Professor of Psychiatry and Behavioral Sciences
University of Washington School of Medicine
Sound Psychiatry Consulting Group
Port Townsend, Washington

Kirk D. Strosahl, Ph.D.

Mountainview Consulting Group Inc.
Moxee, Washington

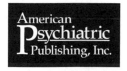

American Psychiatric Publishing, Inc.

Washington, DC
London, England

Note: The authors have worked to ensure that all information in this book is accurate at the time of publication and consistent with general psychiatric and medical standards, and that information concerning drug dosages, schedules, and routes of administration is accurate at the time of publication and consistent with standards set by the U.S. Food and Drug Administration and the general medical community. As medical research and practice continue to advance, however, therapeutic standards may change. Moreover, specific situations may require a specific therapeutic response not included in this book. For these reasons and because human and mechanical errors sometimes occur, we recommend that readers follow the advice of physicians directly involved in their care or the care of a member of their family.

Books published by American Psychiatric Publishing, Inc., represent the views and opinions of the individual authors and do not necessarily represent the policies and opinions of APPI or the American Psychiatric Association.

Copyright © 2005 American Psychiatric Publishing, Inc.
ALL RIGHTS RESERVED
Manufactured in the United States of America on acid-free paper
09   08   07   06   05   5   4   3   2
First Edition
Typeset in Adobe's Garamond and Formata
American Psychiatric Publishing, Inc.
1000 Wilson Boulevard
Arlington, VA 22209-3901
www.appi.org

Library of Congress Cataloging-in-Publication Data
Chiles, John.
    Clinical manual for assessment and treatment of suicidal patients / John A. Chiles, Kirk Strosahl.
        p. ; cm.
    Includes bibliographical references and index.
    ISBN 1-58562-140-4 (pbk. : alk. paper)
    1. Suicidal behavior—Diagnosis.   2. Suicidal behavior—Treatment.   3. Suicide—Prevention.   I. Strosahl, Kirk, 1950–   II. Title.
    [DNLM: 1. Suicide—psychology.   2. Suicide—prevention & control.   WM 165 C537c 2004]
    RC569.C478 2004
    616.85'8445—dc222004050261

British Library Cataloguing in Publication Data
A CIP record is available from the British Library.

Contents

List of Tables

List of Figures

Contributor

Patricia J. Robinson, Ph.D.
Behavioral Health Consultant, Family Practice, Toppenish Yakima Valley
Farmworkers Clinic, Toppenish, Washington

Preface

This book is the result of several decades of spirited debate, friendly repartee, basic research, and clinical collaboration between a psychiatrist and clinical psychologist. Our diverse backgrounds helped us combine training and disciplinary differences to develop a workable approach to dealing with suicidal patients. We hope what has emerged is a valuable, practical approach for clinicians in the field. This book is not meant to be an academic text on suicidal behavior. There are other excellent sources for that. Our goal is to provide you with a sense of what to do with a suicidal patient. The best indicator of our success in this venture is the use of this book in the field, where we hope it will provide clinicians with detailed guidance when working with suicidal patients.

Our discussions and collaborations led us to the decision that it is best to treat suicidal behavior as a method of solving problems. This theoretical stance—that suicidal behavior is problem-solving behavior—is the principle underpinning our approaches to both the assessment and the treatment of suicidal individuals.

We wish especially to thank Patti Robinson, Ph.D. Dr. Robinson is an expert on interventions with those left behind by a completed suicide—the survivors of suicide. Chapter 11, "Understanding and Providing Care to the Survivors of Suicide," is her contribution to this book.

1

Introduction

The Dimensions of Suicidal Behavior

The purpose of this book is to serve as a guide to the individual assessment and treatment of suicidal patients. It also can be used as a training manual. The text, charts, and exercises within each chapter serve as tools for teaching an aspect of the management of suicidal behavior. Our previous publications regarding suicidal patients have been used as training materials, and we have incorporated suggestions from those sources in our chapter design. The use of our earlier materials in China has made us more aware of cross-cultural issues involved in taking on the problems associated with suicidality. Where we can address those issues in this book, we do. We start with five brief case reports—vignettes that demonstrate the multiple forms of suicidal behavior.

Charles D came from an alcoholic family. Heavy drinking had been a multi-generational problem. Mr. D's father, a chronically depressed man whose mood was made worse by frequent drinking bouts, died by suicide when Mr. D was 12 years old. In late adolescence, Mr. D began drinking heavily and, like his father, began to have bouts of depression. Mr. D had frequent

1

thoughts of suicide, ideas that, for years, he shared with no one. At the age of 32, Mr. D married and fathered a child. At age 35, encouraged by his supportive spouse, Mr. D entered psychiatric treatment and within 2 years had no further problem with depression, alcoholism, or suicidal ideation.

Andrea M had been known for most of her life as an individual who quickly displayed a variety of emotions. Her relationships with others were usually intense and often conflictual. Since mid-adolescence, Ms. M frequently talked about ending her multiple frustrations by killing herself. Intermittently, her acquaintances would become concerned and urge her to get into treatment. She never did. As of her 40th birthday, Ms. M continued to communicate suicidal ideation. She never made a suicide attempt.

Ralph H grew up in a single-parent family. His mother worked full-time and reared six children. At the age of 15, Mr. H fell deeply in love with one of his classmates. They dated for a while, and when she ended the relationship, he became very despondent. Mr. H's thoughts turned to suicide, and he decided to end his life. He shot himself in the chest with a 22-caliber rifle. His family rushed him to the hospital, and in time he recovered. Eighteen years later, Mr. H was leading a productive life and was truly glad to be alive. He had no further suicidal ideation.

Mariel R is 34 years old and has been treated for depression intermittently over the past 12 years. In that time, Ms. R has made six suicide attempts, each involving an overdose of prescribed medication. Ms. R leads a difficult life and has frequent and numerous problems. She has multiple worries about her husband's infidelity, her children's illnesses, her employer's behavior toward her, and her finances. Each suicide attempt has been precipitated by an escalation of one of these problems. Ms. R's physician is aware of this history and prescribes antidepressant medication for her only 1 week at a time.

Jose G committed suicide at the age of 76. Before taking a lethal overdose of his heart medication, Mr. G spent 2 days making sure his will was in order. He wrote a lengthy goodbye note to his children and grandchildren. Mr. G led a long and productive life and up to the week of his death had no history of suicidal thoughts or attempts. Mr. G's wife had died 3 months before he committed suicide, he was living alone, and he was experiencing increasing difficulties with the daily activities of life.

Each of these case vignettes demonstrates an aspect of suicidal behavior. Suicidal behavior covers a spectrum of thoughts, communications, and acts.

The least common is completed suicide, death from a self-inflicted injury when there is a determination that the decedent intended to die. More common is attempted suicide, nonfatal self-injury with some intent to die. Most common is suicidal ideation—thoughts of killing oneself.

An important fact to remember about suicidal behavior is how much of it there is. A good deal of the literature on suicidal behavior is focused on completed suicide, the least common behavior. The overall base rate for the United States is relatively stable, at approximately 10.7 deaths by suicide per 100,000 population, or 0.0107% of the population per year. Suicide is the eighth leading cause of death for the general population and the third leading cause of death for individuals 18–24 years of age. Although we are legitimately concerned about death by suicide in late adolescence and early adulthood, we should worry more about the aging population. The suicide rate among the elderly (older than 65 years) is more than double that among those 18–24 years of age. These figures are based for the most part on coroners' reports and may be understatements of the actual suicide rate. Death by accident further confounds the issue. For example, an 18-year-old man dies in an automobile wreck. He was known to be upset over a romantic breakup. While the man is driving alone on a straight road on a clear day, his car plows into a telephone pole, and the man is killed. Friends suspect suicide, the coroner reports the accident, and the truth is never known.

Compared with completed suicide, attempting suicide is a much more common occurrence. Studies designed to establish the frequency of attempted suicide provide variable results—results that seem to depend on the population under study. Asking emergency trauma centers how many attempters they see per year will produce one result, whereas asking a general population sample whether they have ever deliberately harmed themselves with some intent to die will yield quite a different figure. Overall, the lifetime prevalence studies of suicide attempting that we have reviewed vary from 1% to 12%. Our own general population studies, conducted in the greater Seattle area, showed that 10%–12% of adult respondents admit having made at least one suicide attempt.

Suicide ideation, thinking about suicide, is by far the most common form of suicidality. The significance of this ideation can range from a definite intent to die in the context of a severe psychiatric illness (e.g., depression or schizophrenia) to a comforting thought (e.g., if it gets any worse, I can always kill myself). As a colleague once put it, "Thoughts of suicide have gotten me through many a bad night." In our work with general population surveys, we have found 20% of those asked report at least one episode of *moderate* severe suicidal ideation (defined as ideation lasting at least 2 weeks, forming a plan, and identifying the means) at some point in their lives. Another 20% report at least one episode of troublesome suicidal ideation that did not involve formation of a plan. In a more recent study it was found that more than 10 million people in the United States, or approximately 4% of the population, have some degree of suicidal ideation in the course of a year.

In this book, we focus our discussions of suicidality on these three forms: ideation, attempt, and completion. There are many types of self-destructive behavior that may not involve a conscious wish to die. Self-mutilation for the purpose of relieving pain or providing a clear boundary between one's body and the environment occurs in a distinct population. The chronic use of drugs (e.g., alcohol or tobacco) or high-risk behaviors such as race-car driving and mountaineering have been described as a type of subintentional move toward suicide. These behaviors are not the focus of this book but can certainly occur in patients. Treatment of these patients covers a range of psychotherapies and medications, and we encourage reading of that literature to guide therapeutic endeavors.

Although discussions of suicidal behaviors often link ideation, attempt, and completion, suicidality is complex, and there is little evidence that it exists on a continuum. Table 1–1 shows some of the distinctions between the forms. Most people who think of suicide do not go on to make an attempt or die by suicide. Of the 10 million people with suicide ideation each year in the United States, fewer than 30,000 (0.3%) commit suicide. Most people who make a suicide attempt do not ultimately die by suicide. In studies conducted in emergency departments, only approximately 1% of attempters go on to die by suicide in a year. This lack of continuity from one form to another is a key observation from which much of the discussions, observations, and techniques in this book emanate.

Given the prevalence of suicidal behavior and the multitude of causal influences, our conclusion is that suicidal behavior is often designed to solve problems in a person's life rather than to end the life. It is our approach that much of the therapy for suicidality should be based on a learning model— one that teaches new approaches to problems—rather than on a prevention

Table 1–1. Common characteristics of suicidal behaviors in the United States and Europe

Suicidal behavior	Suicide ideation	Suicide attempt	Suicide completion
Sex	Unknown	More among women and girls	More among men and boys
Age	Unknown	Younger	Older
Psychiatric diagnosis	Unknown	50% have no diagnosis	Depression Schizophrenia Alcoholism Panic disorder Comorbidity
Method	Not applicable	Cutting, overdose more common	Shooting, hanging more common

model. Either of these approaches can be used with treatment for a specific diagnosis. Prevention models, predicated in part on the assumption that suicide can be predicted on an individual basis, often rely on three principal strategies. The first strategy is to *emphasize pathology;* that is, to work on the assumption that the suicidal person is experiencing a pathological process, often thought to be depression. The second strategy is to *deliver a maximum response to negative behaviors.* An increase in suicidal behavior prompts a heightened response from professionals that is often centered on the person's weaknesses or deficits. The third strategy is to attempt to decrease suicidal risk by techniques that *lower individual autonomy.* At its most restrictive, this strategy calls for involuntary hospitalization.

A learning-model approach, with less dependence on the assumption that suicidal behavior can be predicted and controlled, alters these strategies. Intervention is focused both on problems that the suicidal behavior is being used to solve and on clinical diagnosis. Efforts are made to focus on the reinforcement of personal strengths in addition to delineation, diagnosis, and treatment of a pathological condition. The clinician's response encourages positive behaviors—the person's unique resources for addressing and modifying the suicidal behavior—as new approaches are found for problems with life circumstances. Efforts to reduce suicidal risk are accomplished by techniques that maximize individual autonomy. A person exhibiting suicidality is assumed to be doing the best he or she can do at that moment to deal with life's difficulties. Our initial task is not to judge or criticize but to acknowledge the struggle and pain the patient has and to begin exploring other ways of dealing with this sea of troubles. Much of this book focuses on developing and finding practical ways to use learning and problem-solving strategies with suicidal patients as they present in a variety of clinical settings.

Can Suicide Be Predicted?

A therapist can claim to have prevented a behavior only if it can be shown that the behavior would have occurred without the intervention. The assumption that suicide can be predicted is a myth in search of facts. It is so important that you understand the ins and outs of attempts to predict suicide that we dedicate a chapter to this topic (see Chapter 3, "A Basic Model of Suicidal Behavior"). However, we will tip our hand early. The tools are not there for making predictions. Although many mental health professionals presume that an important clinical skill is the ability to assess the imminent risk of suicide, this capacity has never been empirically demonstrated. The algebra for such predictive abilities is just not there. In part this problem is base rate in nature because, fortunately, suicide is a rare event. Suicide risk factors are useful in identifying high-risk groups, but they are much less useful in identifying high-risk individuals. In addition, most clinically relevant risk prediction is concerned with the short term (hours to weeks), whereas much of the prediction literature is concerned with the long term (years to lifetime). Furthermore, some long-term risk factors may not be stable. For example, marital status, employment, and current psychiatric diagnoses all can change. In short, on a case-by-case basis our ability to predict either short-term or long-term suicidal risk is markedly flawed. Unless and until significant new risk predictors are developed and evaluated, it is unjustified to assume that a suicide can be predicted. More important, this mistake can lead to the use of less meaningful interventions.

The Role of Psychiatric Diagnosis

Clinicians know, and the psychiatric literature confirms, that suicidality is *not* the province of any one mental disorder. Studies of suicide in different diagnostic categories show suicide death rates consistently ranging from 5% to 15%. Comorbid disorders, especially combinations involving antisocial personality, borderline personality, substance abuse, schizophrenia, panic disorder, and depression, may be particularly lethal. Psychiatric diagnosis has been most emphasized in reports of completed suicide. Suicide attempters are less likely to have a psychiatric condition, and very little is known about the psychiatric state of the multitude of people who have had thoughts of suicide.

Results of several major studies, based in part on retrospective diagnoses and coroners' reports, have shown that approximately 50%–90% of adults who commit suicide have an associated psychiatric disorder. These studies suffer an intrinsic flaw. The dead individual cannot be interviewed, and the recall of others can easily be influenced by the aftermath of a suicide. If you assume that suicide is an indication of a psychiatric illness, you may be more likely to recall events and statements that confirm that assumption. Depression, probably because of its high rate in the general population, is the most frequent diagnosis among those who complete suicide, but the percentage of suicides among the depressed population is about the same as it is among persons with several other mental disorders (e.g., schizophrenia, personality disorders).

Depression poses a particular problem in evaluation of a suicidal person in that it is both overdiagnosed and underdiagnosed. DSM-IV-TR (American Psychiatric Association 2000) lists suicidal behavior as a diagnostic criterion in only one Axis I category: depressive disorders. Perhaps because of this categorization, the two conditions sometimes are equated (i.e., you are suicidal, therefore you must be depressed), and treatment, particularly pharmacotherapy, is started. The diagnosis is based on a series of criteria, not just one. Antidepressant therapy may not be helpful if depression is not the correct diagnosis. Furthermore, some antidepressants (the tricyclics) are quite lethal in overdose and should not be prescribed unless an indication is well established. The rule is simple: Do not *assume* that a suicidal person has a depressive illness, but *always* evaluate for a depressive illness in a suicidal person.

It is now clear that on a national level depression is underdiagnosed. Information from the Epidemiologic Catchment Area studies suggests that more than 50% of people meeting criteria for depression do not receive the diagnosis and are not treated (Sussman et al. 1987). Effective treatments exist, and the effects of treatment on personal productivity and well-being are potentially enormous. Accordingly, all of us need to screen for depression in our evaluations. The best way to do this is to ask patients whether they have ever had a period of 2 weeks or more when they have felt sad, blue, or depressed; have lost interest in things; have lost energy; or have felt hopeless, helpless, worthless, or guilty. If the answer to any of the questions in this brief inquiry is yes, go on to review the criteria for depression. If the diagnosis is established, treat the patient or refer him or her for treatment.

Recognizing and treating psychiatric diagnoses are important and need strong emphasis. However, as we present in many ways in this book, treating the mental disorder is essential but not sufficient for many of our patients, and many suicidal patients (perhaps as many as 50%) do not meet criteria for *any* mental disorder. We recommend that suicidality be treated *in addition to* other treatments administered, and we base this recommendation on two observations. First, many accounts of suicidality have occurred among adequately treated individuals or populations (i.e., suicidal behavior occurred *despite* treatment). In one study the authors (Isometsa et al. 1994) estimated that 45% of suicides occur among patients who are in a treatment relationship with a psychiatrist. Second, effective therapies, particularly pharmacotherapies, have been available for years for major illnesses such as depression, schizophrenia, and anxiety disorders. There is scant evidence that these treatments per se have reduced suicidality in these populations over time. We have substantial evidence from clinical trials that neither antidepressants nor antipsychotic medications are superior to placebo in preventing suicidal behavior (Khan et al. 2000, 2001). The notable exception is the use of clozapine in the treatment of patients with schizophrenia who are suicidal.

Demographic Factors

Most demographic information comes from studies conducted in the United States and Europe. Emerging data from other sources are showing interesting contrasts. For example, although suicide rates are higher for men in the United States, reports from China indicate that women are more at risk to die by suicide. Suicide is more common among the elderly in the United States. The suicide rate increases rapidly among persons 16–24 years of age, plateaus in middle age, and then increases again, in the United States, to more than 20 suicides per 100,000 whites older than 75 years. Most countries reporting suicide rates show that the risk increases with age. Again, cultural differences appear. Suicide rates in later life may decrease among African Americans and Native Americans, most likely because of the low rate of suicide among elderly women in these groups. Suicide attempting seems much more common among the young, there being few reports of attempting, especially first-time attempting, after the age of 45. Although among adolescents the rate of suicide attempts is high relative to the rate of completed suicides (200 or so to 1), the ratio has been reported to be as low as 4 to 1 among the elderly. In the United States, many who attempt do so again. The repetition rate for those hospitalized for attempting is close to 50%. In addition to age and sex, important demographic factors are race, marital status, religion, employment, and seasonal variation. In the United States, suicide is more common among whites. It is more common among the single, separated, divorced, and widowed. Suicide rates may be higher in gay, lesbian, and bisexual groups. Loss of a spouse increases suicidal risk for at least 4 years after the spousal death.

Suicide rates are higher among Protestants than Catholics or Jews, and suicide rates and unemployment correlate positively in many countries. Other factors include the presence of a physical illness, bereavement (based on either recent events or an ongoing reaction to an earlier loss), and physical abuse.

Personality and Environmental Characteristics

In many studies investigators have tried to delineate both personality and environmental characteristics of suicidal patients. Understanding these characteristics is crucial to the treatment model we present. In Chapter 4 ("Assessment of Suicidal Behavior and Predisposing Factors") we spell out the many issues involved. Personality studies, in the main, have been conducted with populations of suicide attempters and ideators and have been focused on four areas of functioning: cognition, emotional distress, interpersonal functioning, and environmental stress. Each of these factors seems important, and the factors probably interact in an interdependent manner. Many cognitive function studies have focused on problem-solving abilities. In general, suicidal individuals have been found to be poor problem solvers. They think in a dichotomous manner, seeing things in terms of black or white, good or bad, right or wrong. A major goal of our treatment approach is to help patients see the gray areas that define most human interactions. Suicidal individuals are both less flexible in their thinking and more passive in the way they solve problems. Much of what they do seems predicated on fate, luck, or the efforts of others. In addition, suicidal individuals often pay scant attention to how often or how well their problem-solving efforts work. They either lack the skills to assess their behavior or do not think about assessment. Without assessment, they are at risk of both choosing and sticking with solutions to problems that either do not work very well or do not work at all. As we spell out our treatment approach, we return to the aspects of personality that affect clinical approaches.

Suicidal patients, the cognitive literature tells us, seem very impatient. They set unrealistically short time lines for success and are apt to jettison a problem-solving solution if it does not produce immediate results. The focus is on short-term gain, and there is often little or no appreciation of long-term consequences. Our work has shown us that many suicide attempters have favorable evaluations of suicide as an effective problem-solving behavior. Moreover, the degree to which they rate suicidal behavior as a problem-solving device correlates quite highly with the seriousness with which they intend to kill themselves. Another important cognitive factor in suicidality is hopelessness, which is predictive of eventual (but not immediate) suicide. The essence of hopelessness is a general sense of pessimism and a feeling of futility about the possibility of life changing for the better. For some individuals, hopelessness may be the link between feeling depressed and then becoming suicidal.

Many suicidal patients are caught in a difficult bind: They have a great deal of pain and have a faulty ability to tolerate it. Their troubled emotional lives are often characterized by anxiety, depression, anger, boredom, and guilt. They dislike the way they feel and have trouble accepting and working with their emotions. They are frustrated, and suicidal ideation and attempting can become a vehicle for discharging pent-up emotion that has no other outlet. Many suicidal patients live in a world of limited social networks and frequent conflict with friends and family. Personal loss and threat of rejection are common, and both are frequent precipitants of suicidal behavior. Suicidal patients often lack competent social support, that is, people who can provide sympathetic and effective help. Incompetent social support consists of people who tend to cajole and lecture rather than listen effectively, support, and teach. Many suicidal patients must deal frequently with the "all you need to do is" form of advice. A metaphor is having a group of religious zealots at the door, each wanting 30 seconds to "change your life." It is difficult for many suicidal individuals to reach out, to form meaningful supportive relationships. New interpersonal situations bother them, and they often suffer social anxiety and withdrawal.

Life stress, both negative and positive, can be a major precipitant of suicidal behavior. Suicidal patients have a high rate of stress, particularly on the negative side. Life for them is a sea of troubles, and daily hassles describe the world of many of these individuals. In addition to having long-term stressors such as physical illness, financial uncertainty, and life-phase changes, suicidal individuals are often beset by a day-in, day-out variety of annoyances. The 24 hours before a suicide attempt is fraught with both minor stress and a high likelihood of interpersonal conflict or loss. Attempts at marshaling support and reassurance from others usually fail, increasing the sense of discomfort and emotional distress.

The Role of Genetics

Genetics plays some role in understanding suicidality. Family history is pertinent to suicidal behavior, but we have more information about completed suicides than about attempts or ideation. Suicide does cluster in families, a finding that suggests a genetic role. Data regarding both monozygotic and dizygotic twins indicate this clustering may represent a genetic disposition to the psychiatric disorders associated with suicide rather than to suicide itself (Roy 1983). The question remains whether there is an independent genetic component for suicide, but suicidality may well be an independent and inheritable risk factor. Genetic influence on other forms of suicidal behavior is much less certain. A family history of suicide does increase the risk of a suicide attempt, pointing to a possible clustering of this behavior within families. We found in our research that suicide attempters are less likely to know other attempters, in their family or not, than are other psychiatric patients or nonpsychiatric control groups. This finding raises the possibility that attempters do not have models that demonstrate longer-term negative consequences of suicidality and are accordingly more likely to see only the short-term, more positive outcomes of their actions. This area is in much need of further investigation.

The Role of Biochemistry

Laboratory work since the late 1970s has been focused on serotonin as it relates to suicidal behavior. Serotonin is a major neurotransmitter, and low levels of this chemical, as measured by its spinal fluid metabolite, are predictive of suicidal behavior in depressed patients. This "low serotonin" observation has been made in other diagnostic groups, including schizophrenia, personality disorders, and alcoholism. Because these findings are made across diagnostic lines, future work may shift the focus of pharmacotherapy for suicidality from depression to a more suicide-specific strategy. Whether medications that target serotonergic function will be helpful in treating suicidal behaviors is a question for further research. In early 2004, the only medication approved by the U.S. Food and Drug Administration for use in the treatment of a suicidal patient is clozapine, and its use is restricted to psychotic illness. In addition, lithium has been shown to reduce death by suicide in populations of individuals with bipolar illness.

The Role of Medical Illness

Medical illness is associated with increased risk of suicide. This association should not be surprising, because the pain, loss of function, disfigurement, and psychological distress that accompany many illnesses can produce problems for which patients may see suicide as a solution. Some serious and chronic illnesses, such as human immunodeficiency virus infection and acquired immunodeficiency syndrome, may be especially associated with death by suicide. It is important, however, to consider suicidality among all severely ill individuals. The presence of a clinically significant mood disturbance in a person with a serious physical illness should always trigger an inquiry about suicidal thoughts. Suicide evaluations are not exclusively the province of mental health professionals. Results of several studies have shown that 50%–75% of persons who commit suicide have seen a physician in the 6 months before death. General health care workers are an important first line of defense in the effort to reduce suicidal behavior.

Conclusion

The psychotherapies developed in the 1940s, 1950s, and 1960s for dealing with suicidality have been at best partially successful. Few preventive treatment strategies for suicidality have succeeded. Little that has emanated from any of the mental health disciplines has had much effect on rates of any form of suicidal behavior. Individuals have been helped, but the problem has persisted. In this book, we do not pretend that we have the answers. We struggle daily with the troublesome concerns of our patients, and, like everyone else, in each case we look for what works best. We are optimistic. We hope individual practitioners can use our book to make their own work more efficient and productive.

Helpful Hints

- Suicidality has several forms, and one form does not necessarily lead to another.
- Nonfatal suicidal behavior is extremely common. The rarest form is completed suicide.

- It is useful to think of suicidality as a method of problem solving.
- Although it is often associated with psychiatric illnesses, suicidality is not necessarily reduced by treatments targeting those illnesses.
- All health care workers are on the front line when it comes to evaluating and initiating treatment of suicidal patients.

References

American Psychiatric Association: Diagnostic and Statistical Manual of Mental Disorders, 4th Edition, Text Revision. Washington, DC, American Psychiatric Association, 2000

Isometsa ET, Henriksson MM, Aro HM, et al: Suicide in major depression. Am J Psychiatry 151:530–536, 1994

Khan A, Warner, HA, Brown WA: Symptom reduction and suicide risk in patients treated with placebo in antidepressant clinical trials. Arch Gen Psychiatry 57:311–317, 2000

Khan A, Khan SR, Leventhal RM, et al: Symptom reduction and suicidal risk among patients treated with placebo in antipsychotic clinical trials: an analysis of the Food and Drug Administration database. Am J Psychiatry 158:1449–1454, 2001

Roy A: Family history of suicide. Arch Gen Psychiatry 40:971–974, 1983

Sussman LK, Robins LN, Earls F: Treatment-seeking for depression by black and white Americans. Soc Sci Med 24:187–196, 1987

Selected Readings

Blumenthal SJ, Kupfer DJ: Suicide Over the Life Cycle: Risk Factors, Assessment, and Treatment of Suicidal Patients. Washington, DC, American Psychiatric Press, 1990

Chiles JA, Strosahl K, Cowden L, et al: The 24 hours before hospitalization: factors related to suicide attempting. Suicide Life Threat Behav 16:335–342, 1986

Conwell Y, Duberstein PR, Cox C, et al: Age differences in behaviors leading to completed suicide. Am J Geriatr Psychiatry 6:122–126, 1998

Crosby AE, Cheltenham MP, Sacks JJ: Incidence of suicidal ideation and behavior in the United States. Suicide Life Threat Behav 29:131–140, 1999

Ettlinger R: Evaluation of suicide prevention after attempted suicide. Acta Psychiatr Scand Suppl 260:1–135, 1975

Hawton K, Catalan J: Attempted Suicide: A Practical Guide to Its Nature and Management, 2nd Edition. New York, Oxford University Press, 1987

Mann JJ, McBride PA, Brown RP, et al: Relationship between central and peripheral serotonin indexes in depressed and suicidal psychiatric inpatients. Arch Gen Psychiatry 49:442–446, 1992

Minino AM, Arias E, Kochanek, KD, et al: Deaths: final data for 2000. National Center for Health Statistics (DHHS Publ No 2002-1120). National Vital Statistics Reports, 50. Washington, DC, U.S. Government Printing Office, 2002

Montgomery SA, Montgomery D: Pharmacological prevention of suicidal behavior. J Affect Disord 4:291–298, 1992

2

The Clinician's Emotions, Values, Legal Exposure, and Ethics

Global Issues in the Treatment of Suicidal Patients

In this chapter we discuss attitudes and perceptions that can strongly shape your approach to suicidal patients and present exercises that will enable you to get more in touch with areas that might pose problems for you. In the first section of this chapter we address the types of emotions that are stirred up by suicidality. In the next section we discuss values and moral reactions in regard to suicide, because your values about suicide and nonfatal suicidal behavior may influence your actions. We ask you to complete exercises that will help you clarify your values in relation to suicide and identify "hot buttons" that may interfere with your ability to work constructively with suicidal patients. Because the fear of lawsuits is a pervasive feature of clinical work with suicidal patients, we take an in-depth look at how civil litigation is structured, the types of legal complaints that are filed after a patient commits suicide, and what you can do to reduce the risk of being sued. Finally, at the confluence of affective response, values, and fears of malpractice is the vital question of how to practice ethically with suicidal patients. We provide a set of guidelines for steering these complicated waters.

Understanding Your Emotional Responses to Suicidal Behavior

Understanding your emotional responses is the first and most important step toward becoming skilled in the treatment of a suicidal person. We start with an imaginary exercise.

Emotions and "Hot Buttons" Exercise

Think first of someone you know who is difficult to understand and somewhat unpredictable. This person is often moody and is intensely involved with other people. Her involvement is often supportive and even flattering, but you have seen it take a dark turn. This person can suddenly, and sometimes for very little reason, become quite angry. The anger is usually transient, but on one or two occasions you have seen it become permanent. This person can turn on a friend and may never speak to that person again. Your own relationship with this person is that of an acquaintance. Your interactions have been social and cordial. Imagine first your feelings about this person as we have just described her. Pause a second, and then imagine that you have just heard that this person has just made a suicide attempt. In the aftermath of the breakup of a stormy relationship, she has cut her wrist, has been rushed by friends to the hospital, and has been admitted to a psychiatric unit. Imagine now what your emotional reaction is. To finish this sequence, you find out that this person has a history of at least three other suicide attempts, one by wrist cutting and two by overdosing. These attempts have been made over 10 years, and all have involved a breakup in an interpersonal relationship. Now think about your emotional reactions to this person. Write each of these emotional responses in the Responses to Suicidal Behavior survey (Figure 2–1). In this exercise we ask you to detail the "best and worst" of you. Record your responses at your emotional extremes. For example, an extremely negative response might be "I would never speak to this person again." An extremely positive response might be "no matter what she does, I will always help her."

Dimension of response	My response	Positive and negative effects on me
What is your primary positive emotional response?		
What is your primary negative emotional response?		
What aspects of this person's situation and behavior elicit the most negative or judgmental response from you?		
What aspects of this person's situation and behavior elicit the most positive or compassionate response from you?		
What is the biggest barrier you would encounter continuing to interact with this person?		

Figure 2–1.   Responses to Suicidal Behavior: first survey.

Now imagine a different person, a friend from your childhood. This person is now in his mid-40s and has had a rough time of it for the past 3 or 4 years. His two teenage children have been troublesome, and one, a daughter who has been failing in school, has recently been arrested for drunk driving. This person's spouse has become increasingly withdrawn from the marriage and has made many trips to various doctors because of physical ailments, none of which has been identified with any particular illness. Six weeks ago, your friend was laid off from his job. Imagine your emotional response to this person. Pause. Now imagine your response to learning that he has made a suicide attempt. This past weekend he was drinking heavily, something that he hardly ever did. Late Saturday night this person shot himself in the chest with a handgun. This person's family rushed him to the hospital, and he is now in serious but stable condition. Imagine your emotional response to hearing of this person's suicide attempt. Write these responses on a second Responses to Suicidal Behavior survey (Figure 2–2).

Once you have thought about both your positive and your negative responses, make a change. Think of each of these individuals as patients of yours. Each has been in treatment for 3 months, at which point each makes a suicide attempt. Does this change your responses? Does the nature of the relationship make a difference in your emotional responses? Are you more tolerant of suicidal behavior in acquaintances or in patients? If so, why is your response different on the basis of the type of relationship you have?

Last, think about the persons just described, but make one more change. Rather than hearing that each has made a suicide attempt, you have learned that each has committed suicide. Think of your emotional responses at this point and write them down. Are your responses different when you are faced with fatal versus nonfatal behavior?

Evaluation of Responses

Most of us have strong reactions to acts of nonfatal self-destructive behavior, suicidal ideation, and suicidal verbalization by others. We tend, however, to feel and behave differently when dealing with a completed suicide. Passivity and philosophical resignation are often present with suicide. In contrast, suicide attempting, ideating, and verbalizing have powerful and often negative emotional pull. In describing patients who manifest these behaviors, clinicians unfortunately tend to use a variety of highly charged phrases, such as "he

Dimension of response	My response	Positive and negative effects on me
What is your primary positive emotional response?		
What is your primary negative emotional response?		
What aspects of this person's situation and behavior elicit the most negative or judgmental response from you?		
What aspects of this person's situation and behavior elicit the most positive or compassionate response from you?		
What is the biggest barrier you would encounter continuing to interact with this person?		

Figure 2–2.   Responses to Suicidal Behavior: second survey.

is a manipulator," "that was only a suicide gesture," or "that is typical behavior of a borderline personality." These statements can cause difficulties in working with an acutely suicidal patient. If you have not dealt with your capacity to have these "gut level" responses, their negative impact will most likely arise in the midst of a suicide crisis—in other words, the worst possible time. The clear thinking required could become muddled at precisely the moment when it is most needed.

Recall now your emotional responses to the cases described earlier in the emotions and "hot buttons" exercise. In the first case, a typical response on hearing about the suicide attempt may be that it made some sense; it fit the way that person was leading her life. You may have felt some concern but also some relief that you were not the person involved in the chaotic relationship that set it off. You may have felt some anger at the person for using suicidality in a "manipulative" way. A typical reaction to learning that there had been multiple suicide attempts would be to find your rejection of the patient increasing, to feel increasing relief at not being involved, and to feel wariness about having much to do with this person in the future. What did you feel when the situation changed and the person completed suicide? Many people would feel passivity, resignation, and some sadness, often accompanied by the feeling that there was a lot more happening than one knew about.

Many people find it easier to relate to the person in the second case. So many rotten things were going on that the emergence of suicidality is understandable. Adding the weekend bout of alcohol abuse makes it even easier to both have a sense of the situation and begin to think of solutions. In this man's case, we might be less likely to become angry or irritated and more likely to have a sense of both "yes, I understand that" and even "there but for the grace of God go I." Imagine that 3 years have passed and you have lost contact with this person for some time. He recovered from the gunshot wound and left the hospital. You learn not only that the drinking continued but also that your friend had been quietly drinking too much for years and had frequently been verbally abusive to his wife and children. Since the gunshot wound, this person has made three other suicide attempts, all by overdosing. The overdosing has been done with antidepressants, because he has been in some form of treatment for some time. This person has divorced, lives alone, is still out of work, and is still drinking. He has just contacted you and asked for a loan, stating, "If you can't help me, I don't know what I will do." What is your emotional response at this point?

There is even a more difficult side to our reactions. It involves the value we place on our ability to heal and the reduction of that ability in the midst of a suicidal crisis. Most health and mental health providers go into the profession because they like to help people. Their tandem assumption is that patients seek these services to be helped. However, a suicidal patient may be ambivalent about being helped, and this ambivalence can seriously impair treatment. In this situation, clinicians are reminded that both their healing authority and their powers of persuasion are limited. When persuasion fails, clinicians get in touch with their powerlessness, and they have to deal with it. In this situation, many of us experience frustration and anger, and if we are not careful, we may blame these emotions on the patient's behavior. We can feel off balance and begin to react to, rather than treat, our patients. Interactions can begin to center on the patient's ambivalence and negative attitudes rather than on the work that needs to be done. What can surface is a showdown over conformity, and the patient's potential for suicidal behavior is in the center of the struggle. In these moments, we can, unfortunately, challenge the patient to "put up or shut up," to either play by our rules or seek help elsewhere. Whatever the outcome, the working relationship is over—as much because of our issues as because of the patient's problems.

Morals- and Values-Based Stances on Suicide

An exercise that we have found very helpful in workshops is to discuss the various values people hold about suicide—often based in philosophies that have evolved over several thousand years—and express almost every possible point of view. In many societies throughout history, suicide has been the focus of philosophy. The stances range from statements about suicide being unequivocally wrong to statements that suicide is an intrinsically positive act. What follows is a summary of this spectrum of approaches. Each approach has its adherents, and arguments about validity (or lack thereof) can be made about each point. Read through these, and think about your own philosophy. At the end, we will tell you ours.

Suicide has been described as an unequivocally wrong and harmful act. It can be viewed as doing violence to the dignity of human life, as something against basic human nature. A philosophy that reveres every human life, in which it is felt that life should be preserved at all cost, is at its foundation opposed to suicide. In a religious context, suicide can be seen as a wrongful consequence of pride, usurping God's prerogative to give and take away human life. Suicide can be seen as homicide and thus forbidden. A more socialistic philosophy may indicate that suicide is wrong because it represents a crime against the state. In this scenario, a person would be described primarily as a social being, the property of the state. No person has the right to deprive the state of its property. Suicide has been described as unnatural. When a person commits suicide, violence has been done to the natural order. From a more psychological perspective, suicide can be seen as wrong because it presents an oversimplified response to a complex and necessarily ambivalent situation. It is an irrevocable act that denies future opportunity for learning and for growth. From the viewpoint of systems psychology, suicide can be seen as wrong because it adversely affects the survivors, both the immediate family and the general community.

Bending somewhat from the unequivocal wrongness of suicide, one could think of suicide as permissible under certain conditions. This philosophy would support the suicide of a person who has no opportunity for quality of life. A person dealing with a painful, incurable, and lethal illness, for example, could justifiably commit suicide. Suicide may be viewed as an issue without moral or ethical overtones. Suicide has occurred across cultures and across time and is a phenomenon of life that is subject to scientific study much as any other phenomenon may be. Suicide can be seen as an act that takes place beyond the realm of reason. Suicide can occur by motivations that are unintelligible to the rational mind but justifiable on the basis of mystical experience. Suicide may be a morally neutral act. Every person, through the right of free will, can make or take his or her life.

Just as a number of philosophies have evolved that describe suicide in a negative way, a number have evolved that describe it in a positive way. For example, Epicurius stated that the purpose of life is enjoyment (Dewitt 1954). When pleasure ceases, death becomes a comfortable and available alternative. In some cultures, suicide is viewed as a reasonable choice. Death can be considered a lesser evil than dishonor, and suicide can be encouraged—a preference for self-destruction rather than defeat. Some cultures use suicide as a way of dispensing justice. For example, tribal law that prohibits incest might be enforced by requiring anyone breaking this law to leave the tribe and kill himself. Justice would thus be restored. Suicide might be a permissible act when it is performed for some great purpose, for example, self-immolation in the cause of peace. Suicide might save face when a person is perceived to have lost honor. Suicide might be a positive way in which one can immediately reunite with valued ancestors and with loved ones. At times, suicide has been presented in a personified and eroticized manner, a poetic expression of both beauty and the seductiveness of death.

Let us examine your personal values and moral stance on suicide. Each of us through our upbringing, life experiences, and personal struggles has developed a set of beliefs about the act of suicide. The important thing to realize about values is that they can never be proven; as humans, we just acquire them. Another important feature of values is that they drive our behavioral, evaluative, and emotional responses. Therefore it is extremely important for you to thoroughly understand your attitudes about suicide. Do you see suicide as a wise choice sometimes? Does it make you angry? Is it a difficult and troubling topic for you to talk or think about? If after reviewing these various philosophies you feel some trouble or concern, talk it over with your colleagues. Seek counseling for yourself if you feel that would help. Before you see your next patient, get a good handle on how you feel. The worse time to have to deal with this issue is when your patient is in a crisis.

To see where you stand, we recommend that you complete the values and moral response self-assessment that constitutes Appendix A (Philosophies About Suicide) and then analyze the results. Do you see yourself endorsing beliefs that are negative toward the act of suicide? This attitude may lead you to be overly moralistic in your approach to a suicidal patient. Do you endorse a mixture of negative and positive beliefs? That might suggest that you are ambivalent or conflicted about your stance toward suicide. There may be clinical situations in which you could sympathize with a patient's desire to die, whereas in other situations you may not be so sympathetic. For many of us, our philosophies are not stable but tend to change depending on the circumstances with which we are dealing. We urge you to assess yourself, because you must decide whether you can comfortably work with suicidal individuals. There is nothing right or wrong about having a temperament and a point of view that make such work very difficult, if not impossible. Your work is a matter of inclination and type of talent. If working with suicidality is not for you, then do not do it. It is far better to deal with this issue now than when you are asked to treat an acutely suicidal person, a person to whom you have made a commitment to treat.

More Self-Examination

Two instruments we use to evaluate suicidal patients are found in Appendix B (Consequences of Suicidal Behavior Questionnaire) and Appendix C (Reasons for Living Inventory). These questionnaires are included because we would like you to complete them as part of the process of self-examination.

Consequences of Suicidal Behavior Questionnaire

The Consequences of Suicidal Behavior Questionnaire (Appendix B) is another exercise of the imagination. Before starting the questionnaire, put yourself in a suicidal frame of mind and then list some consequences of your suicide attempt and your completed suicide. We cannot give you much information about how to imagine that you are suicidal. For some of us the affect would be hopelessness, for others anger, and for others anxiety. Likewise, the problems that precipitate suicidality vary. For some it would be a massive and overwhelming difficulty. For others a series of long-term, daily hassles. You have to create this frame of mind for yourself. If we knew, in some universal sense, what caused suicidality, then the field would have made a major advance.

When you have completed the Consequences of Suicidal Behavior Questionnaire, go back through your results. How closely do your answers correlate with your values and moral stance in relation to suicide? Did you see any good in the consequences of your attempted suicide? For example, would other people become more focused on helping you? Would your problems become more apparent, both to you and to others, making help that much easier to obtain? What about bad results? Does embarrassment or loss of face play a role in your reactions? Did the results of your suicide attempt tend to be all bad or all good? Go back to the exercise and try to produce some more results, this time in a direction different from that of your original consequences. By doing this exercise, you will get a sense of both the complexity and the ambivalence of the suicidal crisis. Another factor to look at in your attempted suicide results is the nature of the problems you listed. First, did you list any problems? It is our contention that suicidal behavior is problem-solving behavior. If most of your answers relate to how you or other people feel, revisit your responses. Look beyond the statement of feeling to a statement of problem. Feelings must be dealt with and can block successful treatment. *Always* look past the feeling for the problem being addressed.

A second part of the Consequences of Suicidal Behavior Questionnaire involves the completion of suicide. Are there religious or philosophical overtones to your sense of what happens to you after death? Is it easy to come up with two different results, or is it hard? For many of our patients, even those who have thought long and hard about suicide, we have found that the spectrum of potential consequences has not been examined. The suicidal patient de facto sees things as being better after death whether or not an afterlife concept is present. Many magazines have stories about "near-death" experiences that are positive and peaceful in overtone. This aspect of death tends to be the sole consequence with which the patient is in touch. If the patient generates results that are bad, an antisuicidal effect may occur. Another dimension of the exercise is the importance or unimportance of individual consequences of your suicide. Some consequences of suicide that seem to be universally important (e.g., effects on children left behind) may be rated as unimportant by a patient. Check the consequences of suicide that you feel are important and unimportant and compare them with those of your friends and colleagues. What are the similarities and differences? Return to the exercise and try to come up with two more results that have a degree of goodness and importance that are different from your first ones. This step will help you think through the ambivalence and complexity of suicidality.

The questions concerning those left behind have been raised to force an issue. When a person is expressing suicidality, these aspects are seldom thought about. You probably found it fairly easy to think about survivors. In imagining suicide, it is not hard to come up with effects on survivors. In general, doing this exercise will dampen your ardor for your imagined suicide. Look back at the two case examples in the emotions and hot buttons exercise. A good part of your emotional response to the suicidal patient could come from your concern about the consequences to the survivors. You are on the outside looking in and can see the effect on those left behind. When you are on the inside, when you are the suicidal person, it is much more difficult to think about your survivors.

The last part of this exercise involves comparing your reasons for committing suicide with the reasons others give. What reasons did you conjure up for yourself, and do they differ from the reasons you attribute to other people? Most important, do your reasons for committing suicide differ from those you attribute to other people who attempt suicide but do not die? Many of us assign different sorts of reasons to the actions of those who attempt suicide. Often these reasons suggest that the attempt was manipulative and based on weakness of character. The reasons of others seem less important than those that we would attribute to our own imagined circumstance. This line of thinking can color your emotional reaction to suicidality. If you find the reasons varying in these three sections, come up with additional reasons. Most successful therapists have the ability to put themselves in their patients' shoes, to see the world, as sympathetically as possible, as their patients see it. Use this exercise to test your limits for that ability.

Reasons for Living Inventory

The Reasons for Living Inventory (Appendix C), the other exercise in this section, has to do with the positive side of suicidal ambivalence, the answers to why I want to stay alive. In Appendix C, the inventory has been arranged to show six dimensions. Ask yourself the following question: If I were thinking of suicide, what are the reasons I would have for *not* killing myself? Now read through the inventory with that question in mind. Is your sense of being able to survive and cope important? What is your responsibility to your children or to other family members? Does the act of suicide scare you, such that this fear becomes a reason for avoiding suicidal behavior? How do you feel about social disapproval, the fear of "losing face"? Last, what are your moral objections, if any? After taking inventory of yourself, go back to the two case examples in the emotions and hot buttons exercise or to other examples that you may have generated from your own experience. Think about how those two suicidal persons would answer this scale. More than that, answer this scale for them, make them as real as possible and get a sense of how much they would agree or disagree with each question. Has your affective response to this person changed as a result of your answers? It probably has, because you have just expanded your view of the patient. You may have come up with a way of assigning the patient some positive attributes. Furthermore, you have new tools for a therapeutic discussion and probably feel more comfortable about your ability to engage with a suicidal person.

The lesson learned with these exercises is of universal importance in dealing with suicidality and reflects a practical philosophy about suicide. As a clinician, always try to understand the totality of patients' views of suicide and then reinforce the positive side of suicidal ambivalence. Make the following

assumption: "This person is talking to me because of ambivalence about suicide. If there is an unequivocal desire to commit suicide, this person would
probably already be dead. My job is to find the spark of life that brought the
person here and reinforce it." Our philosophy is this: Suicide is one way of
solving problems, but there are usually better ways.

Legal and Risk Management Issues

The industrialization of mental health services has had enormous benefits for
patients who previously had little or no access to behavioral health care. However, this transformation from a "cottage industry" to "service industry" has
been accompanied by an increased risk of malpractice litigation. Clinicians
who in the early part of their careers practiced with relative immunity from
malpractice claims now find themselves compelled to review the legal and risk
management implications of their clinical decision making on a daily basis.
Malpractice insurance is a prerequisite for any practitioner who wants to provide behavioral health services. Larger institutions such as psychiatric hospitals and mental health centers have risk management departments whose staff
includes attorneys who specialize in both interpreting the risk associated with
clinical services and devising protocols for minimizing the civil and criminal
risks associated with such services. When an adverse event such as a patient
suicide occurs, not only is the clinician left to cope with the anguish of losing
a patient but additionally the clinician may have to answer to a plaintiff's attorney, a judge, and a jury. In response to the increasingly litigious nature of
the health care environment, many texts and journal articles have been intro-
duced to articulate both clinical and legal standards for providers who have
medical training and those who do not. The Selected Readings list at the end
of the chapter contains some of the better books and articles on this subject.
A defining feature of legal standards of care is that they are derived from the
outcomes of malpractice litigation. This practice constitutes an ethical danger: Standards of care derived by jury verdicts may have minimal overlap with
what the science states is evidence-based care. Between us, we have more than
50 years of experience working as expert witnesses in both civil and criminal
proceedings related to suicidal deaths. The purpose of this section is to ac-
quaint you with the anatomy of a lawsuit, the types of negligence claims that
are at the basis of most lawsuits, and ways in which you can protect yourself

from being sued. Keep in mind that there is no "silver bullet" that will immunize you against a lawsuit. However, understanding the process of civil litigation may alert you to basic safeguards that will prevent you from being an "easy mark."

From Adverse Event to the Courtroom

A 42-year-old man is referred by family members to a psychiatrist for counseling because of increasingly frequent talk about killing himself. He is going through a messy divorce and reports that he has been drinking two to four beers per night to help calm himself down. He reports that he has little social interest and mainly spends his time at home ruminating about the impending divorce. He indicates that his thoughts frequently turn to vivid and specific images of loading his handgun, putting it in his mouth, and pulling the trigger. He reports feeling a greater sense of peace when thinking about suicide. He reports that he does have a handgun at home, and it is loaded. He reports that 5 years ago, after a particularly bad marital dispute, he took an overdose of 3 aspirin tablets but drove himself to an emergency room before any physical damage occurred. He realized at that time that he did not want to die. Now he is not so sure. He reports that he has tried everything he can think of to feel better but believes that most of his subsequent efforts to correct his life will fail.

After making the diagnosis of severe depression, the psychiatrist initiates a phased-in prescription of trazodone 300 mg/day. A no-suicide contract is secured from the patient, and the patient agrees to give his guns and ammunition to a neighbor. This action is confirmed by the patient at the next visit 3 days later. The psychiatrist feels at this time the patient need not be involuntarily committed. The patient does not want to be hospitalized and reports feeling somewhat better. Vegetative signs of depression are improving. A third appointment is scheduled for 3 days later. The patient calls and cancels the appointment, stating he is going back to work. He accepts a new appointment 5 days later. On the phone, he reports feeling much better; vegetative signs are much improved. That night, the patient does not return home, and his wife calls the psychiatrist, who recommends that she contact the police. The next morning the patient is found in his pickup dead from a gunshot wound, the gun having been purchased the day before. The widow sues the psychiatrist and the associated physicians group, claiming that the patient should have been involuntarily hospitalized, that the psychiatrist should not have accepted a no-suicide contract from a patient with a mental disorder, and that the psychiatrist should have made contact with the patient's friends and family about the treatment plan. Her case is that each of these actions or omissions failed to safeguard the patient, causing the suicide.

Most practitioners do not realize that there is a considerable time lag from the time of an adverse event such as a patient suicide to the filing of a negligence claim. We have found a delay of 2–4 years is not at all unusual. Typically, in the case of a suicide, the bereaved survivors may be too grief stricken to pursue litigation for months, or even years. At this emotional level, they may even be ambivalent about filing a lawsuit. It generally takes a long time for a plaintiff to decide to become a plaintiff.

The time lag between a suicide and the filing of a negligence claim has many practical implications. First, most clinicians have "moved on" from the adverse event until they receive the notice that a claim has been filed. They may not remember many of the specifics of the case or the immediate circumstances that prevailed at the time of the patient's death. Because of these factors, the clinician must rely extensively on written documents, such as intake reports, progress notes, medication summaries, and discharge summaries. Thus the quality of these documents and their content is critical to a defense in a lawsuit.

Second, the lag between the occurrence of a tragic event such as a patient suicide and the decision to file a lawsuit suggests that there may be opportunities to intervene with the survivors of suicide in a way that may short-circuit their decision to seek civil remedies. At the psychological level, a lawsuit can be a systematic attempt to prove that someone other than the survivor is to blame for a patient's suicide. Working through the sense of guilt and responsibility is a key theme in clinical work with survivors of suicide. If this process goes awry, the decision to file a lawsuit may be the result. Our experience suggests that many civil negligence lawsuits are induced by the reactions of the providers and institutions involved. For example, one psychiatric hospital was sued as a direct result of billing a suicide survivor for the psychiatric inpatient treatment of a spouse who committed suicide in the inpatient unit.

Third, most clinicians are thunderstruck when a patient commits suicide, and it may take many months to resolve feelings of guilt and failure resulting from the conviction that somehow the provider failed to deliver appropriate care. By definition, if that care had been delivered, the patient would not be dead. Being drawn back into a review of one's professional competence after putting these issues to rest is quite traumatic. Once this Pandora's box is re-opened, the providers involved see the lawsuit as a chance to be vindicated— only to be bitterly disappointed when their insurance company reaches an out-of-court settlement.

Finally, it is important to realize that the Anglo-American system of law is a faulty system of justice. The ability to procure effective legal representation, the characteristics of the presiding judge, the composition of the jury, and the sympathy factor are all important elements of a law proceeding. Much like behavioral health, most of the outcome in lawsuits is determined by nonspecific factors. Juries in particular are highly variable in their application of the law. As the O.J. Simpson trial suggested, anything can happen once the jury is out.

Malpractice Claims

The typical scenario is that a plaintiff's attorney within a local or regional jurisdiction files a negligent death claim. The claim has to establish a set of facts about the process of care that transpired before the suicide. In the claim the plaintiff tries to demonstrate how the actions of one or more providers were negligent. The typical claim usually is organized chronologically, starting with the first providers and services that were delivered that are alleged to be part of the causal chain. The claim then lists each allegation of negligence provider by provider and event by event. The claim ends with a request that the court award the plaintiff monetary damages. Monetary damages usually are awarded separately for the loss of likely lifetime earnings of the decedent and for pain and suffering and loss of companionship on the part of the survivors. It is important to understand that the case itself is fought not only on the negligence claim but also on the amounts of lost earnings capacity and actual pain and suffering experienced by the survivors.

In most lawsuits, the most common strategy is to create a list of negligent acts—a simple application of probability theory that is widely used by plaintiffs' attorneys. The more negligent actions one alleges, the greater is the likelihood that the judge or jury will agree with at least one allegation. The more numerous and outrageous the claims, the more likely it is that a jury will conclude that some malfeasance had to occur to generate that many complaints. A similar litigation philosophy is used to name defendants. A plaintiff's attorney usually names several defendants, at both the agency and individual provider levels. The more defendants named, the greater is the likelihood that at least one will be found guilty of a negligent action. On a practical level, naming more defendants activates more liability insurance policies, which increases the pool of funds that can be drawn from if a settlement is reached. Three to five defense attorneys may be involved in a typical suicide negligence lawsuit, and each of these attorneys has a separate charge from a different insurance company to defend.

Once an insurance company is notified that a patient suicide has occurred or becomes involved as an insurer for a provider who has been sued, a very specific process is initiated that most health care providers do not understand. If the patient has committed suicide but no lawsuit has been filed, the insurance company immediately conducts an internal review of the specifics of the case with the aim of quantifying the risk of a successful malpractice suit. This internal review typically is not subject to subpoena. After this review is completed, the insurance company identifies an adverse-event loss figure. This number is the amount of money the company estimates it may have to spend in attorney's fees, travel expenses, expert witness fees, and the likely award to the plaintiff if the jury believes that a negligent death has occurred. This figure is supposed to be a closely held secret, but a skillful plaintiff's attorney can generally determine the loss reserve on the basis of responses received during settlement discussions.

It is important to know that most lawsuits never make it to trial, because most insurance companies believe it is in their best interest to reach an out-of-court settlement. Some behavioral health providers are shocked to discover that their liability insurance policy has a provision that requires the provider to participate in a reasonable settlement as determined by the insurance company. Failure to do say may result in the insurance company's refusing to pay subsequent attorney's fees or to pay a malpractice award. If this situation sounds like big business at work, it is. The civil litigation industry is a multi-billion dollar enterprise involving the transfer of great sums of money between the legal and insurance communities. Unfortunately, an out-of-court settlement is viewed by most state licensing authorities and behavioral health credentialing systems as a successfully prosecuted action against the licensed provider. Without ever admitting guilt, the provider is viewed as guilty. Before agreeing to a settlement in a wrongful death suit, defendants should make sure they understand all of the licensing and credentialing implications of the settlement.

The Process of Discovery

Discovery is a general term used to describe the process of fact finding that leads to one of three outcomes: 1) an out-of-court settlement is reached; 2) the judge delivers a "summary judgment" that effectively decides the lawsuit, usually for the defendant; or 3) the judge orders the case to go to trial. There are two major components to the process of discovery, and it is important to understand them both.

The *interrogatories* are a process designed to make sure that all records, tests, personal diaries, and any other documents that may have bearing on the case are available to all parties. These documents are instrumental in helping the court determine whether negligence occurred and how to adjudicate the subsequent financial award. Interrogatories are bidirectional. Either side in a lawsuit can make extensive requests for this type of information. Practitioners involved in a lawsuit can expect to produce all pertinent patient care records, including such items as original session notes, correspondence with other practitioners, phone records, and billing records, to name a few.

An important part of the interrogatory process is the production of expert witness reports, which are evaluations of whether the defendants involved in a case met or did not meet the standard of care. Both sides usually hire expert witnesses to review all data pertinent to the case and then render a set of opinions about whether negligence was involved. Not surprisingly, the experts for the plaintiff nearly always describe the defendant's care as negligent, and the defense experts maintain that the care provided by the defendant was well within the standard of care.

Although every state has a legal definition of standard of care, the job of the expert witness is to persuade the jury what the standard of care actually is. For this reason, an expert witness typically is a provider in the germane discipline—in this case has acknowledged expertise with suicidal patients. Often this expertise is established by producing a record of publications, presentations, or training sessions in the area of suicidal behavior. Functionally, two types of experts are involved. One is an expert in the subject area, in this case, suicidal behavior, even if the expert's discipline is different from that of the defendants. The second type of expert is a provider in the same discipline who testifies about the standard of care for that discipline. This type of expert may have no particular expertise in the arena of suicidal behavior but is used to establish what would be expected from a competently trained provider in the same discipline. In nearly every suicide lawsuit, the attorneys employ both types of expert witness.

The other major component of the discovery process is the taking of depositions. The overall goal of the deposition process is to provide each side with a complete information set. In effect, each side is attempting to "discover" in advance what a witness is going to say on the stand. A deposition is a court-ordered process that involves obtaining information about the case from various witnesses under oath. Depositions usually are obtained from all plaintiffs and defendants, expert witnesses, family members and friends of the decedent, economists, and any other person who may have information bearing on the facts of the case. Testimony given in a deposition can and will be used in the trial portion of a lawsuit. For the defendant in a suicide lawsuit, the deposition can be a harrowing experience. The plaintiff's attorney not only digs relentlessly for information but also tries to get the defendant to provide conflicting answers to questions, to second-guess his or her clinical care, and to admit under oath to one or more of the negligence claims made in the original legal claim.

The Civil Trial

Assuming that the presiding judge has not issued a summary judgment, the trial phase begins with the selection of a jury. The composition of a jury is just as important in a civil suit as it is in a criminal proceeding. Attorneys take a good deal of time interviewing prospective jurors in an attempt to qualify or disqualify them. This phase is also the attorney's opportunity to form a positive relationship with each juror, who may later sway other jurors over to a more favorable verdict. In many respects, however traumatic the trial phase is for the defendant, it is really an anticlimax. Very little new information is presented at a trial. The intensity of the discovery process usually brings most of the facts of the case to light before the courtroom proceedings begin. Each side attempts to highlight the facts and opinions that support their point of view. The major difference between a civil and a criminal trial involves the standard of evidence required to deliver a verdict. Civil law uses a standard called a *preponderance of evidence.* This standard requires that the majority of the evidence suggest that negligence did or did not occur. This "preponderance" could be as small as 51% to 49%. In contrast, criminal proceedings use the standard of *beyond a reasonable doubt,* meaning that there should be no doubt that the defendant is guilty.

The civil standard for returning a verdict is so much more lenient than the criminal standard that it was possible for O.J. Simpson to be acquitted of murder in criminal court and then be found guilty of wrongful death in the subsequent civil proceeding. In many states, juries are required to allocate responsibility for an outcome between the plaintiff and defendant. For example, the jury may conclude that the plaintiff was 70% responsible for committing suicide and the defendant contributed 30% to the outcome. The allocation then determines how much of the award amount is the responsibility of the defendant and the plaintiff. Typically, juries are more bimodal in these allocations. In other words, they are likely to award 90% to the plaintiff or 95% to the defendant rather than to "split the pie." The rationale is that any allocation to the defendant represents an award to the plaintiff whereas the opposite relationship does not hold.

Characteristic Claims in Wrongful Death Suits

The first step in managing your legal risk is to understand the kinds of negligence complaints that are typically contained in civil suits resulting from a suicide. Malpractice is defined as a pattern of negligent or willful misconduct on the part of the behavioral health provider. The burden of proof is on the plaintiff to show that the negligence was the result of a lack of knowledge, skill, or care that would ordinarily be exercised by a similarly trained provider under similar circumstances. Furthermore, the plaintiff must prove that the defendant's lack of knowledge, skill, or care was the proximate cause of a death that otherwise would not have occurred.

Several assumptions are contained in this rather standard definition of malpractice. First, there is a commonly accepted standard of knowledge, skill, or care that should be exercised by any competently trained provider. Second, negligent actions can be errors of omission or of commission. Errors of omission are actions that should have been taken but were not. Errors of commission are inappropriate or badly misguided actions. Third, there is the concept of a pattern of negligence or willful misconduct. Negligence is very hard to prove on the basis of a single error. A pattern of errors leads to the determination of negligence. Fourth, willful misconduct implies that the provider deliberately engaged in negligent or substandard care. Willful misconduct generally is unlikely to be the claim in a wrongful death suit unless financial or personal motives are suspected. Perhaps most important, the concept of proximal cause means that a direct and uninterrupted link exists between the last in the pattern of negligent acts and the death.

Because negligence can involve both errors of commission and errors of omission, it is useful to examine the kinds of claims that are made in a negligent death suit. In truth, a wrongful death lawsuit is an exercise in 20/10 hindsight. A competently trained provider never engages in every single action that is cited in a negligent death suit. In the hypothetical world of law, the endless number of levels of analysis leads to a type of infinite regress.

Inappropriate or Inadequate Assessment

In almost every case, the plaintiff tries to prove that the practitioner made an incomplete or inappropriate assessment of the patient's suicidal risk and failed to properly judge other clinical factors that might contribute to suicidal potential. An incomplete assessment is an error of omission. An inaccurate assessment is simply drawing a badly misguided conclusion about the level of suicidal risk. With regard to the assessment of suicidal risk, typical problem areas are the alleged failure to assess the remote or immediate history of suicidal behavior, failing to properly evaluate current suicidal potential, and failing to corroborate with significant others information obtained from the patient. If the provider has documented a suicide risk assessment, the plaintiff will claim that the provider drew the wrong conclusion on the basis of the omission of other contributing factors in the clinical decision-making process. Contributing factors might involve not asking about current drug or alcohol abuse and failing to adequately diagnose depression or some other life circumstance known to dramatically increase emotional distress and suicidal tendencies.

Failure to Hospitalize or Treat Aggressively

The most common claim in this arena is that the patient should have been hospitalized rather than treated as an outpatient. If the patient was treated as an inpatient and then released, the claim will be that the patient needed additional inpatient care and should not have been released. If outpatient care is part of the suit, the claim will be that session frequency and between-session intervals were insufficient to constitute a meaningful response to the patient's level of suicidality. When a suicidal patient has canceled an outpatient treatment session, the claim will be that the provider should have seen this as a sign of increased suicidal risk. These claims are made even in cases in which the ostensible reason is actually evidence of a positive treatment response (e.g., the patient has returned to work and needs to reschedule the therapy appointment).

Failure to Refer for Consultation

Most often, the claim of failure to refer for consultation involves the decision of a provider who does not have medical training to treat a suicidal patient without the use of a medicine that might have been indicated. Another claim is that the provider should have sought a psychiatric consultation to determine whether the patient should be hospitalized.

Failure of Communication Between Providers

If more than one behavioral health provider is involved in the patient's care (e.g., a social worker and a psychiatrist), a common claim is that not enough information was shared between the providers and that the second provider underestimated the patient's real suicide risk. Another claim is the failure of two providers to communicate on a predictable basis, leading to one provider's but not the other's being aware of the emergence of a new risk factor. In inpatient suicide cases, the most typical complaint is that various hospital staff failed to communicate essential information in shift-change briefings or that one or more staff members had access to patient information that was not effectively communicated to shift supervisors and other hospital staff.

Failure to Reassess Suicidality

Many suicides occur well into the treatment process, rather than immediately after the initial visit. The typical claim is that the provider failed to reassess the patient's suicide risk and to establish a revised treatment plan at every visit. Another common claim is that the provider failed to involve family members and other informants so that they could provide additional information about the patient's suicidality over time.

Failure to Follow Patient Protection Protocols

Failure to follow patient protection protocols is a common malpractice claim made in hospital-based suicides. One typical claim is that the "suicide precautions" level was not intensive enough given the patient's degree of risk or that the required line-of-sight observation of the patient did not occur according to hospital policies. If the patient was placed on suicide precautions and then moved to normal status, the challenge will be that the decision to go to normal status was inappropriate. In nearly every hospital suicide case, there is a claim that the hospital has failed to provide adequate continuing education to all staff in the assessment and treatment of suicidality.

Failure of Facility Safeguards

The most common complaints involve the inadequacy of suicide protections in the design of inpatient units. For example, a floor plan that leaves the nursing station out of line of sight of the restraint and seclusion room might be cited as the cause of a suicide while the patient was in seclusion. Another lawsuit will claim that the failure to install breakaway showerheads in patient rooms is the cause of a death by hanging from a showerhead. Yet another negligence claim might focus on the security of window locks if a patient has picked the lock and jumped.

The Search for the Elusive Standard of Care

A key determinant of the outcome of a malpractice suit is how the "standard of care" will be defined for the jury. This is the linchpin for determining whether the defendant is guilty of negligent practice. *In most states, the standard of care is legally defined as the care that would have been exercised in similar circumstances by a similarly trained provider in the community at the time the alleged negligent action occurred.* It is important to realize that the crux of the contested nature of a lawsuit is that both sides will try to establish a different standard of care. The defendant's legal team will portray the defendant's care in the most positive possible light. The plaintiff will try to do the opposite.

Ultimately, the jury will reach consensus on what the standard of care was at the time of the adverse event.

There are several important implications of this definition of standard of care. First, the adequacy or inadequacy of professional care is established with reference to a provider in the same discipline. If a psychologist is sued, the standard of care is defined by what a similarly trained psychologist would do under similar circumstances. In other words, different standards are used for determining negligence, depending on the discipline of the provider. Social workers, psychologists, marriage and family counselors, and psychiatrists are held to unique standards of care. In lawsuits in which more than one provider is named, the jury may be asked to form opinions about several distinct standards of care.

Second, standard of care is a hypothetical concept that is developed on a case-by-case basis. A textbook on standards of care of suicidal patients may be produced as an authoritative source but in and of itself cannot conclusively establish the standard. In general, expert witnesses produced by the defendant and plaintiff have the greatest influence in helping a jury derive a standard of care.

A third implication is that the standard of care can vary from locality to locality. A provider in a remote rural community may not have access to a psychiatric facility, and the general practice in that community may be to deliver care that does not require the use of a psychiatric facility.

Finally, the standard of care may vary according to the date of the adverse event. In general, a defendant cannot be held accountable for delivering a type of care that was not generally available in the community at the time of the suicide. A new and more effective treatment may have appeared after the adverse event, but negligence cannot be determined with respect to what was not a common clinical practice at the time of the event.

What Is the Standard of Care for the Treatment of Suicidal Patients?

In clinical practice with suicidal patients, it is important to adopt a general treatment philosophy that will withstand the rigors of an intense legal examination. The following definition provides the type of guidance that would generalize to almost any mental health setting and would place any provider in good position in the event of a lawsuit:

> The standard of care requires the mental health provider to collect enough relevant information during the initial and return appointments to estimate the patient's mental status, establish relevant mental health diagnoses, properly understand the patient's current functioning, and finally, to use this information to arrive at an assessment of the patient's relative risk for self-harm. The provider must use this information to determine whether it is clinically appropriate and safe to continue treatment in the outpatient setting. If the patient is a minor, the provider's duties are to collect information from both the patient and parents or guardians, to accumulate a reasonable history, to compare the minor's and the parents' points of view, and to corroborate important information.

Protecting Yourself From Lawsuits

Every practicing clinician needs to understand that the risk of a lawsuit goes hand in hand with being a mental health professional. There is no foolproof method of preventing lawsuits, just as there is no magic solution for the problem of suicide. The things that can go wrong in clinical treatment of a suicidal patient are too numerous to mention; however, the best medicine for protecting oneself from, and preparing oneself for, a negligence lawsuit is fairly direct. The following guidelines are not derived from the precedents set in civil lawsuits but rather reflect the contributions of clinical common sense, scientific inquiry, and ethically sound practice.

Conduct a Competent Clinical Assessment and Document the Plan

Good clinical practice involves conducting a reasonably thorough initial assessment of the patient's suicidal behavior. Even if the goal is not to predict a suicide, it is always useful to conduct at least a brief suicidal behaviors assessment. In Chapter 4 ("Assessment of Suicidal Behavior and Predisposing Factors"), we provide tools for conducting such assessments and interpreting the results. Suicidal behaviors assessment should usually include a review of past suicidal behavior, recent suicidal ideation or behavior leading up to the patient's seeking therapy, and a review of the patient's beliefs about the efficacy of suicide as a problem-solving strategy. This assessment can be done in a way that is direct, matter of fact, and not terribly time consuming. It is reassuring to patients struggling with suicidal thinking or behavior to see a therapist approaching these behaviors in a nonalarming, straightforward way. Without writing a book, it is important to document in the patient's chart what the suicidal behaviors assessment reveals and how this information will be addressed (or not addressed) in the treatment plan. If the decision is to continue with outpatient treatment or to involve family members in some way, make sure this plan is written in the chart. Mental health providers are paid to make clinical decisions based on their professional judgment. The legal risk of being found guilty of malpractice is much less likely when the data leading to a clinical decision are clearly documented, even if the outcome is adverse. The most common problem encountered in the courtroom is incomplete documentation of what assessment data were collected, how these data led to the clinical decision that was made, and how the data were converted into a treatment plan. Remember this legal mantra: *If it is not written in the chart note, it did not happen.*

The following sample chart note may serve as a guide in documenting treatment:

> John M returns today for a 50-minute follow-up appointment. Continues to report some depression, with insomnia, loss of appetite, and significant anhedonia. He states he is taking his antidepressant as prescribed and has been following his behavioral activation plan (exercise ×3 weekly; two social contacts weekly). He reports that his mood is improved since the initiation of treatment. He indicates he has had episodes of suicidal ideation over the last several days but denies any suicide attempts. He reports that these episodes are brief and sporadic and that he generally "bounces back" within 15–20 minutes. On a 1–10 scale of severity, he rates the worst episode a 4, but more generally they are 2–3. He denies any current intent to engage in self-destructive behavior. States he does not see suicide as a solution to his problems. On the basis of this information, I do not feel he is at risk of self-destructive behavior at this time and is most appropriately treated on an outpatient basis. We reviewed the crisis response plan that will allow him to call me or the emergency services unit should his functioning deteriorate. Plan is to return in 1 week for 1:1 outpatient treatment.

Seek Informed Consent

It is always useful to seek informed consent at the first contact and document what was discussed with the patient in terms of treatment options, risks and benefits, agreed-upon protocols for addressing suicidal emergencies, and the patient's choices regarding selection of various treatment alternatives. This process does not have to be onerous, but it helps to offset any notion that the patient or significant others were not allowed to participate in the treatment-planning process. In a fairly high percentage of negligent death lawsuits, plaintiffs claim that the patient and significant others were not fully informed about the various treatment options available and that they were not educated about the risks and benefits of each option. Inpatient hospitalization, in particular, is one treatment alternative that is the subject of such claims. Documentation of the treatment alternatives discussed and what was agreed to by the patient, significant others, or both is a very good countermeasure for the pervasive problem of selective recall once a lawsuit has been filed.

Reassess Suicidal Behavior Over Time

If a patient enters therapy with suicidal behavior as a presenting problem or develops suicidality over the course of treatment, it is important to periodically reassess the suicidal behavior at each session. Again, this process does not have to be a time-consuming, nerve-wracking "risk management" exercise but is simply an open, matter-of-fact attempt to collect data about the patient's status since the last session. If there is a change in the patient's status, note the change and any clinical decisions that are made. It is important to remember that the appearance or reappearance of suicidality is not an automatic indication that the treatment is not working. In other words, if the impression is that the patient is working in therapy, then the treatment plan may not need revision. If the treatment plan is revised (e.g., additional sessions are scheduled), note the revision in the chart. Remember that the chart note will often be the best method for recalling what care was given and why, if a legal challenge is made.

Document Peer Review and Professional Consultations

If a suicidal patient is discussed in an interdisciplinary team meeting, document that fact and any "core feedback" that might be important to the treatment plan. Even when an interdisciplinary group agrees wholeheartedly with a treatment plan, this consensus should be noted however briefly in the chart. The standard of care does not require a therapist to seek peer review or second opinions, but use of these avenues and documentation of their use in the chart create the impression that the provider practiced cautiously and deliberately. When a patient is referred to another provider for a second evaluation, note the rationale for the referral and include either the second provider's consultation note or a summary of the feedback. Although it can be a bonus in terms of impression management in a lawsuit, seeking consultation can be a disadvantage if it appears that the provider did not integrate the second opinion into the treatment process. Again, proper documentation provides the "ounce of medicine" that is needed.

Make Evidence-Based Treatment Decisions

In the development of a treatment plan, it is often helpful to include a sentence or two about how the scientific evidence supports the treatment that is being delivered. For example, if the decision is to treat the suicidal patient on an outpatient basis, the provider might note that the evidence suggests the best outcomes are likely to be achieved using that modality instead of an inpatient modality. Providers who show a commitment to delivering treatments that are supported by science generally impress members of a jury. Expert witnesses generally try to impress jurors with the same type of tactic, so it is a positive strategy to behave as an expert in documenting evidence-based treatment rationales.

Do Not Be Fooled by Suicide Prevention Measures

It is worth repeating one more time: No interventions have been shown to prevent suicide. A paradox is that suicide prevention strategies such as no-suicide contracts can lull a provider into believing that the level of suicide risk has been substantially reduced when in fact it has not. Use of a prevention strategy may decrease the likelihood that the provider will maintain the proper level of vigilance around increasing suicide risk. We have been involved in several cases in which patient suicides occurred soon after the "successful" implementation of classic suicide prevention strategies. If the decision is made to use such interventions, the measures should always be regarded as interim and time-limited strategies. A no-suicide contract made at session one is not necessarily still in force at session two. Some lawsuits have focused on the fact that a suicide prevention strategy is initiated but then is not reviewed and reaffirmed at each subsequent contact. In general, if they are going to be used at all, prevention interventions should be documented at each session. Again, prevention measures are not "treatment," but they may be part of an integrated treatment plan.

Reduce Policy- and Procedure-Driven Services

One of the paradoxes of civil negligence is that a provider or agency can be found negligent simply for failing to follow agency policies and procedures, even if those policies incorporate clinically useless strategies for treating a suicidal patient. Thus, a provider can dramatically exceed the typical standard of care and yet be found guilty of negligence for violating agency policies and procedures. There is danger in codifying too many risk management strategies into practice standards. These policies become the de facto "standard of care" in relation to a claim of negligence. The plaintiff will claim that the policies constitute a separate "standard of care" that can be applied to any clinical employee covered by the policy. In general, it is advisable to keep the number of required clinical interventions to the minimum. Instead, craft risk management policies and procedures so that they are evidence based and emphasize the singular role of clinical judgment in determining the specific interventions called for. For example, an agency policy that requires inpatient hospitalization for a patient who refuses to sign a no-suicide contract is simply an invitation to a plaintiff's verdict. It is better to describe a range of factors that may or may not contribute to a clinical decision to hospitalize a patient.

Risk Management After the Index Suicide

When hearing of the suicidal death of a patient, most mental health providers enter into a state of emotional shock and disbelief. In most cases, the suicide is an unexpected event. In the midst of this turmoil, it is important to remember that the behavior of the providers and the responses of others in your agency or clinic can have a considerable impact on the likelihood of a subsequent lawsuit. In addition to immediately notifying the liability insurance carrier of the adverse event (allowing the carrier the opportunity to conduct a risk management appraisal of the case), you should also try to use the following guidelines.

Reach Out to the Survivors

It is simply a humane and ethical act to make contact with the immediate survivors of the deceased patient and to invite them to participate in some form of grief counseling. Either the therapist of record or another provider may conduct counseling, but the recommendation is to try to connect the survivors with the therapist of record. An attempt should be made to have the survivors enter into a longer episode of counseling such as a local "survivors of suicide" group. If an agency is involved, the agency should make every effort to allow the survivors immediate access to all records pertinent to the patient's care. Any effort to sequester records from survivors will automatically generate suspicion that the provider or agency is hiding something. The survivors should be relieved of all financial responsibility for clinical services predating the suicide attempt. This outreach response should be immediate, unequivocal, and nondefensive. These responses tend to engender sympathy from the survivors, who realize that the providers involved with the patient are also in a state of shock and grief.

Never Alter the Clinical Record After the Fact

If a patient commits suicide, providers should avoid the temptation to alter existing chart notes (often to specifically mention that they had assessed the patient's suicidal risk in the last session) or to add new chart notes containing retrospective analyses. In a state of shock, some providers begin the process of soul-searching by analyzing the process of care in the patient's chart. This analysis may include comments about what the provider thinks he or she "missed" or reflection on clinical strategies the provider should have used. In some circumstances, these notes have incriminated other providers who may have had a role in the treatment of the patient. In general, it is important to be cautious about what goes in a patient's chart after suicide. These chart notes are very difficult to explain in court, and they may not only discredit the patient's primary provider but also provide ammunition for incriminating other providers.

Never Second-Guess a Decision

Once an adverse event like suicide has occurred, it is always easy to imagine what could have been done differently in the course of clinical care. This line of thought is, in fact, the "trump card" of the plaintiff's attorney. Again and again, the attorney will return to the question of what the provider should have done differently. The more you are willing to acknowledge that different assessment or treatment strategies would have produced a better outcome, the more the stage is set for a determination of negligence. In this situation, it is important to remember that there is no evidence that suicide can be predicted or prevented in an individual case. Thus the use of different assessment or treatment strategies would not improve the likelihood that the suicide would have been prevented. In deposition and on the stand, you have to stand tall and basically say this: Given the information that was available at the time and given my clinical training and experience with suicidal patients, it is highly likely that I would draw the same clinical assessment and engage in the same treatment plan. If presented nondefensively, this type of response convinces jurors that the provider reached clinical decisions that, given the information at hand, were clearly within the standard of care.

Although it is inherently absurd to assume that a self-inflicted act such as suicide can be *caused* by the actions of another, this assumption is "reality" as defined by the U.S. legal system. In the final analysis, the legal system is based on the interpretation of broad statutes. One way to begin reducing the volume of litigation is to sponsor laws that better define what types of psychiatric outcomes can by definition be incorporated in negligence claims. Defining suicide as self-inflicted death that cannot be predicted or prevented would much more accurately represent the nature of the act itself and specifically honor the fact that the mental health profession does not currently possess the technology needed to prevent such deaths.

Ethical Issues in the Treatment of Suicidal Patients

Many clinical suicidologists maintain that it is the duty of every therapist to prevent a patient from committing suicide. Unfortunately, doing so is easier said than done. Furthermore, the extent to which this "requirement" supersedes any of our other ethical obligations to a patient is far from clear. Some providers argue that the duty to preserve life legitimizes any number of actions, however invasive they may be (e.g., breaching confidentiality, involuntary hospitalization). At the level of clinical practice, this black-and-white ethical stance grossly oversimplifies the complexities of any particular patient's life circumstance. We do not mean to suggest that legal and ethical standards must necessarily conflict. We do mean that the application of ethics in clinical practice is not a simple matter. With the growing influence of legal fears, a clinician may not be able to easily differentiate what is ethically indicated from what is legally indicated. If you do not maintain awareness of these divergent influences, you can end up enforcing the interests of the society to the detriment of the patient. The interpretation and application of ethics in these circumstances is an entirely subjective exercise, even when colleagues are called upon to provide guidance. Ultimately, ethics are not played out in the lofty presence of philosophers, priests, and ethicists. Instead, they are applied in the "trenches," where the analytical picture is cloudy, human suffering is great, and the clinician must respond as much from the gut as from the head.

Ethical standards are living, breathing principles that must be put to the test of "workability." Workability means that whenever an ethical dilemma is encountered, the goal is to do the right thing for the patient, regardless of pressures to go in a different direction. Workability represents the basic paradox in applying ethics to clinical work with a suicidal patient. We must learn to be aware of our legal, agency, and risk management responsibilities without becoming trapped in them. Does the legal requirement provide useful guidance, or does it result in a patient's being damaged even though the "correct" risk management procedures have been followed? Who is being protected in this situation—the patient, the therapist, or the interests of society? Is the law being applied to hide what amounts to your negative moral or emotional response toward the patient? What should be done when the law and professional ethics suggest conflicting courses of action? Each of these questions will surface more than once in a career of working with suicidal patients.

Ethical Guidelines for the Treatment of Suicidal Patients

All therapists are required to adhere to ethical standards within their discipline. Almost always, the first rule is to administer no harmful treatment. *Primum non nocere*—"First, do no harm"—was pronounced by Hippocrates millennia ago. Harm, in the case of working with suicidal patients, originates in two main areas: 1) interference from personal reactions, morals, and beliefs about suicide and 2) failure to use assessments and treatments that have been shown to work. We briefly review these two areas of harm and suggest some general guidelines for you to follow.

Ethically speaking, it is your duty to make sure that your emotional responses, moral or religious beliefs, and personal values about suicidal behavior do not cloud the process of selecting and implementing treatment strategies that are in the patient's best interests. In one instance, the therapist may believe that suicide is an individual choice that should not be restricted by legal sanctions. In another, the therapist may believe that by contemplating suicide, the patient has sinned against God. Both stances can produce destructive effects if they are allowed to intermix with therapy in an uncontrolled manner. The more permissive therapist may not work as hard to find alternatives to suicide as a way to solve the patient's problems or may subtly grant the patient permission to complete the act. The antisuicide therapist may engage in blaming, moral lecturing, confrontation, and threats of incarceration in a state hospital.

The solution to this dilemma is simple in concept, complex in practice. The therapist must attend to the patient's beliefs, moral evaluations, and perspectives on suicide; work to create additional alternative solutions for the patient; and not confuse personal beliefs with those of the patient. These goals can best be met by following some specific guidelines.

First, you should regularly inventory your morals and values about the issue of suicide and nonfatal self-destructive behavior. Morals, values, and emotional reactions to suicidal behavior can and do change with maturation and specific life experiences. It is critical to periodically check in with one's moral beliefs to detect any change from previous self-assessments. We suggest that you assess your morals and values concerning suicidal behavior by reviewing Appendixes A–C (Philosophies About Suicide, Consequences of Suicidal Behavior Questionnaire, and Reasons for Living Inventory) at least once a year.

Second, you must determine whether your emotional response, morals, or values preclude you from being able to treat suicidal patients. There is no shame in concluding that your reactions to a particular clinical problem make it very difficult or impossible to work effectively with patients who have that problem. It is better to acknowledge this up front than to engage in ineffective or even destructive treatment. When you are in doubt, it is often useful to talk these issues over with a colleague who may be able to provide much-needed perspective.

Third, the therapist should communicate directly and nondefensively with the patient about the issue of suicide. This interaction is tantamount to obtaining informed consent from the patient about your approach to treating suicidal behavior. The ideal situation is that the exchange results in a mutual exchange of beliefs about suicidal behavior. This interaction should include a discussion of the types of treatment available, the risks and benefits of each treatment, and an attempt to engage the patient in the process of treatment planning. In essence, this ethical requirement amounts to seeking the patient's informed consent to treatment.

Fourth, the therapist must make it clear to the patient what he or she is prepared to do if the patient engages in suicidal behavior or presents with suicidal risk. This discussion includes the conditions in which the therapist may call for emergency medical care, seek to have the patient hospitalized, or be willing to receive crisis phone calls from the patient.

Finally, you must make it clear that the job of therapy is to help people find the best possible solutions to life's difficulties. The therapist should clearly communicate hope that the patient will not commit suicide and should make it clear to the patient that no assistance will be rendered to help the patient commit suicide.

A second standard most of us strive for is to use only effective treatment approaches. A terribly misguided concern is present in some therapists because of their desire to first do no harm. The concern is that if you ask about suicidal behavior, you may be planting a suggestion in a vulnerable person, and he or she will go on to engage in such behavior. No clinical experience or research findings support this assumption. Asking about suicidality is the first step toward treating suicidality. This fear has been particularly expressed about children and adolescents, who are seen as more vulnerable to the power of suggestion. Again, there are no data that in any way support this assumption. In fact, the harm comes from *not* asking about suicidality. At best, you will miss important information. At worst, you will leave your patients with a sense that this is a taboo topic and is a problem for which they can expect no help.

A dedication to using only effective treatment approaches is an ever-present but all too often ignored ethical standard. The problem comes when the documentation for the effective treatment is still lacking. Parenthetically, this is a problem for a variety of human ailments. To date, there is little in the treatment literature about suicidality that substantiates the clinical utility of existing inpatient or outpatient treatments. Often the therapist is aware that the treatment is not working but has no good alternatives. Sometimes the therapist is convinced that a particular treatment strategy would work, only to find that agency policy and procedure do not allow that strategy. We have seen several examples in which systems dictate procedures regarding suicidal risk management that providers believe to be at best ineffective and at worst bad for the patient. An example is an insistence on hospitalization for everyone voicing suicidal ideation or for patients who refuse to sign a no-suicide contract. This discomfort over the feeling that current interventions are not working and needed interventions are not available is a major ethical dilemma. The frustration arising from this dilemma, if not dealt with directly and appropriately, can lead to a bad outcome. Sessions can deteriorate into lecturing, pleading, or confrontation about suicidal behavior. None of these techniques works very well; in fact, these techniques may harm the patient by fracturing the working alliance. The therapist may start secretly hoping that the patient will not show up for the next appointment and may begin behaving in a variety of ways that will give that message. The patient can feel equally frustrated. Once again, things are being talked over, and not much is happening. For some patients, this scenario is an unfortunate repetition of an experience they have had many times before.

There are several ways to minimize ethical dilemmas. First and foremost is to remember that the intervention is designed to help the patient. At regular and agreed-upon intervals, ask whether the treatment is helping. If not, ask the patient what needs to be done to make the sessions more helpful. Put aside your defensiveness; you are not omnipotent, and you may not be on the right track with this particular patient. Refer the patient to another provider if both of you agree that would be more helpful.

A second way to avoid ethical problems is to stay abreast of developments in the field. This knowledge maximizes your chances of being effective, even within system constraints. It is also important to use what you learn to build up an internally consistent approach. The more you believe in your approach, the more effective you will be with it.

Finally, it is becoming increasingly clear that systems as well as providers are going to be held accountable for policy-based interventions. If you work in a system that has policies that guarantee ineffective or harmful treatment, you need to gather peer support and attempt to change these policies. Remember, if a policy is rubbing you the wrong way, the great likelihood is that it is doing the same to others. The "quality of care" protest, especially when formalized in writing and signed by several staff members, is a very effective device for bringing about change.

Helpful Hints

- If you are not aware of your emotional reactions, moral or religious response, and personal values about suicidality, you will not treat your patients in a logical and consistent manner. Use the exercises contained in Appendixes A through C (Philosophies About Suicide, Consequences of Suicidal Behavior Questionnaire, and Reasons for Living Inventory) to become aware of your own "hot buttons."
- You must have practice strategies in place that help protect you from the risk of malpractice litigation without having your fear of lawsuit dominate your treatment approach. Complete the exercise in Appendix E (Malpractice Management Assessment) to see where you stand in this regard.
- Ethical practice with suicidal patients involves keeping your personal reactions to suicide and your legal fears in check while you pursue an evidence-based approach to working with suicidal behavior. You should not engage in treatment options that lack scientific support, even if they are called for in agency guidelines.

Reference

Dewitt NW: Epicurius and His Philosophy. Minneapolis, MN, University of Minnesota Press, 1954

Selected Readings

Bongar B: The Suicidal Patient: Clinical and Legal Standards of Care. Washington, DC, American Psychological Association, 1991

Bongar B, Berman A, Maris R, et al (eds): Risk Management With Suicidal Patients. New York, Guilford, 1998

Gutheil TG: Paranoia and progress note: a guide to forensically informed psychiatric recordkeeping. Hosp Community Psychiatry 31:479–482, 1980

Linehan M, Goodstein J, Nielson S, et al: Reasons for staying alive when you're thinking of killing yourself: the Reasons for Living Inventory. J Consult Clin Psychol 51:276–286, 1983

Litman RE: Psycholegal aspects of suicide, in Modern Legal Medicine, Psychiatry, and Forensic Science. Edited by Curran W, McGarry AL, Petty CS. Philadelphia, PA, FA Davis, 1980, pp 841–853

Murphy GE: Problems in studying suicide. Psychiatr Dev 1:339–350, 1983

Nolan JL (ed): The Suicide Case: Investigation and Trial of Insurance Claims. Chicago, IL, American Bar Association, 1988

Perr IN: Suicide litigation and risk management: a review of 32 cases. Bull Am Acad Psychiatry Law 13:209–219, 1985

Robertson J: Psychiatric Malpractice: Liability of Mental Health Professionals. New York, Wiley, 1998

3

A Basic Model of Suicidal Behavior

In this chapter we provide you with a simple, effective, and clinically useful way of thinking about suicidal behavior. Our focus is on suicidal behavior as a learned method of problem solving that involves escaping from or avoiding intense negative emotions. A secondary effect of suicidal behavior is that it is a very effective way (intentionally or unintentionally) to change one's environmental situation. The near universality of suicidality suggests that this behavior cannot properly be thought of only as a sign of a mental disorder, although it certainly is increased in a variety of mental disorders. However, many patients with mental disorders such as depression, schizophrenia, and panic disorder do not report suicidal ideation, nor do they make suicide attempts. Equally important is that many people who think about, attempt, or complete suicide do not have a mental disorder. If the presence of a mental disorder does not fully explain why a patient becomes suicidal, what additional information do you need to have a comprehensive framework from which to build a complete treatment program for your patients? A serious psychopathological condition must be recognized and treated in its own right, but we are convinced that other clinical factors are more basic determinants of whether an individual engages in suicidal behavior. Dealing with suicidal behavior as a distinctive set of behavioral predispositions, apart from the role played by the presence or absence of a mental disorder, is likely to make you more effective in your treatment approach. In essence, we are asking you to look beyond the diagnostic label the patient carries and assess how this patient deals with emotional suffering. We believe that this approach will help explain why so many people engage in suicidal behavior across age groups, across diagnostic categories, and across a variety of troublesome life situations.

Figure 3–1 shows a multidimensional model of suicidal behavior. The model is derived from a review of the research literature. It has been confirmed in our clinical experience with a wide range of suicidal patients over the last decade. This model emphasizes four important components that collectively predispose a person to suicidal behavior:

- Intense negative emotional states created by problematic internal or external events or triggers
- A passive problem-solving style characterized by escape and emotional avoidance strategies and an inability to tolerate high levels of distress
- A learned, reinforced pattern in which thinking about suicide or attempting suicide is associated with short-term reductions in distress
- A paradoxical increase in negative emotional arousal that results from using suicidal thinking and behavior as a form of emotional control

The Role of Problems

Suicidal behavior seldom occurs in a vacuum. Patients usually are confronted with internal states or external events that are extremely difficult for them to handle. Internal states are negative feelings, such as depression, anxiety, loss, fright, unremitting boredom, anger, or any number of other unpleasant affective experiences. Usually there are external problems in the patient's life as well. For example, severe feelings of loss or guilt may be triggered by a marital separation or impending divorce. Anger may be precipitated when a patient has been betrayed or undermined by someone who was counted on as a friend or support. The patient may have a chaotic, stress-filled lifestyle that involves many daily hassles or the day-to-day problems that can drive one to distrac-

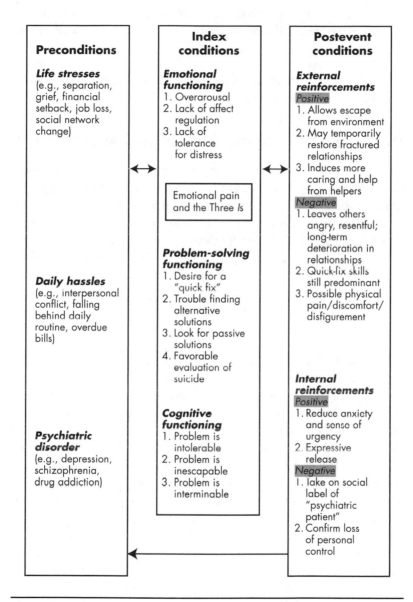

Preconditions	Index conditions	Postevent conditions
Life stresses (e.g., separation, grief, financial setback, job loss, social network change)	**Emotional functioning** 1. Overarousal 2. Lack of affect regulation 3. Lack of tolerance for distress Emotional pain and the Three *I*s	**External reinforcements** Positive 1. Allows escape from environment 2. May temporarily restore fractured relationships 3. Induces more caring and help from helpers Negative 1. Leaves others angry, resentful; long-term deterioration in relationships 2. Quick-fix skills still predominant 3. Possible physical pain/discomfort/disfigurement
Daily hassles (e.g., interpersonal conflict, falling behind daily routine, overdue bills)	**Problem-solving functioning** 1. Desire for a "quick fix" 2. Trouble finding alternative solutions 3. Look for passive solutions 4. Favorable evaluation of suicide	
Psychiatric disorder (e.g., depression, schizophrenia, drug addiction)	**Cognitive functioning** 1. Problem is intolerable 2. Problem is inescapable 3. Problem is interminable	**Internal reinforcements** Positive 1. Reduce anxiety and sense of urgency 2. Expressive release Negative 1. Take on social label of "psychiatric patient" 2. Confirm loss of personal control

Figure 3–1.   A problem-solving model of suicidal behavior.

tion. These problems often accumulate, and one particular daily hassle may function as the proverbial straw that breaks the camel's back. The underlying theme is simple:

• Suicidal patients are always experiencing significant emotional pain, regardless of the source of such pain.

The Role of Emotional Control and Avoidance

A broad literature indicates that there is a strong relationship between emotionally avoidant coping styles and a variety of psychopathological conditions (Hayes et al. 1999). Furthermore, results of studies of problem-solving skills in suicidal patients suggest that these patients rely on passive strategies such as luck, changes in the behavior of others, or simply the passage of time. Together, the tendencies toward emotional avoidance and reliance on passive strategies constitute a very tenuous "gasoline and a match" psychological state.

What do we mean by emotional avoidance? Simply put, emotional avoidance means that rather than making room for or accepting emotional pain, the patient attempts to control, eliminate, or suppress the negative experience. Most of us are trained to believe that negative emotional states are bad (toxic) and that something must be done about them—that the goal of living is to feel good and that bad feelings are indicative of a mental illness, lack of character, lack of willpower, or some other negative personal attribute. The natural tendency is to look for solutions or coping strategies that can eliminate these bad experiences so that we can return to the default state of feeling good again. This outlook means the goal of coping with a life dilemma is to eliminate the bad feelings it produces and develop good feelings. This line of thought is the normal change agenda that suicidal patients bring into the office. When negative emotional states cannot be deliberately controlled (as is always the case), the patient turns to more and more extreme forms of behavior to gain control. More extreme forms of emotional control are almost always quick acting and carry marked negative consequences over time. This method of coping may explain some aspects of the high comorbidity between suicidal behavior and alcohol and drug use, eating disorders, addictive behaviors, and self-mutilation. These behaviors are birds of a feather. They are quick-acting attempts to eliminate or control negative affect. The key component of this part of the model of suicidal behavior is as follows:

- Suicidal behavior is an extreme form of emotional avoidance. It is exhibited to gain control over unwanted feelings, thoughts, memories, or physical sensations. Although it is active in its self-destructive modalities, the behavior itself is a passive way of solving problems.

The Role of Learning and Reinforcement

The idea that suicidal behavior is learned means that it is shaped and maintained by reinforcements. Reinforcement is an event that occurs before or after the suicidal behavior that either rewards it or punishes it. A reward is something that encourages more of a behavior. A punishment is something that promotes less of a behavior. Suicidal behavior is shaped by rewards and punishments. Shaping means changing a behavior so it receives maximum rewards and minimum punishments. The development of a suicidal coping style is the result of the reinforcements that occur in proximity to the behavior. Suicidal behavior, once it is shaped, is maintained. The concept of maintenance means that suicidal behavior will remain so long as it continues to receive reinforcement. When all reinforcements are removed from the behavior, it will be extinguished (i.e., it will disappear). Let's examine how this process works.

Just as suicidal behavior is a response to internal or external problems, the reinforcements are also internal or external. Internal reinforcements involve changes in one's physical, mood, or mental state. For example, reduction in anxiety or fear is an extremely potent internal reinforcement. Many suicidal patients report a sense of relief after making a suicide attempt. The anxiety over whether self-destructive urges can be controlled is gone, even though suicidal behavior has occurred. After the attempt, thinking about suicide or making a suicide attempt is looked at as a way to relieve the terrible sense of anxiety and internal pressure at the heart of an emotional crisis. The goal of eliminating, suppressing, or controlling negative emotional experience has been achieved.

External reinforcements are events that occur in the world as a response to an individual's suicidal behavior, and there are many of them. Several external reinforcements are shown in Figure 3–1. Among those shown, the most important positive reinforcements are increased attention and caring from loved ones and (not infrequently) mental health providers. Furthermore, this behavior pattern can produce very elementary environmental shifts that might help the patient address primary needs such as hunger and shelter. In addition, the patient can escape from what are often chaotic and conflicted living situations. The main principle to apply in treatment is as follows:

• Suicidal behavior is a learned coping response and problem-solving strategy. This behavior pattern can produce a range of fairly dramatic effects on internal mood states and environmental stressors. These effects can make suicidal behavior a very effective short-term problem-solving behavior.

The Role of Short-Term Versus Long-Term Consequences

To understand how suicidal behavior is learned and why it persists, one must appreciate the difference between short- and long-term consequences. A short-term consequence is an immediate effect of suicidal behavior. The time frame can be minutes to several days. Anxiety relief is a very short-term consequence; it occurs within minutes or seconds of the suicidal act. The goal of immediate emotional control is always a short-term consequence. If the only thing that matters is obtaining relief from immediate emotional distress, then suicidal behavior is a very effective response.

An intermediate or long-term consequence may take weeks, months, or even years to develop. These consequences develop in the domains in which the problem-solving behavior originated: internal and external. Internally, we encounter a paradox that results from the use of suicidal behavior to regulate emotional pain. The attempt to control emotional pain actually makes emotional pain stronger. Why is this so? Emotions cannot be regulated through artificial acts; they can only be temporarily numbed. When these emotions return, the psychology of the situation changes dramatically. The emotions have to be compensated again, this time by a more serious version of suicidal thinking or behavior. The patient is caught in a strange loop. The more suicidal thinking or behavior is used to quell the original emotions that were unwanted and unacceptable to the patient, the more powerful those same experiences become. A race is run between the patient's escalating suicidality and the escalation in negative affect.

In the external world, we see a similar paradoxical effect. The intimate others of the patient will initially respond to suicidal behavior with a quasi-compassionate response that may appear to signal a change in the way relationships are going to be conducted. However, what can and often does develop is anger and resentment over the coercive nature of this forced reconciliation. Whereas the short-term consequences of suicidal behavior are very often powerful and positive, with other people appearing to become concerned and sympathetic, the long-term consequences produce a paradoxical rebound effect whereby intimate others come to feel used and manipulated. However, when the immediate change agenda is emotional control, the long-term effects are secondary to the immediate mission: out with the bad feelings, in with the good feelings. Evaluated in this light, suicidal behavior is an extremely potent problem-solving behavior.

It is important to emphasize suicidal behavior as a legitimate form of problem solving. In the patient's mind, suicide can be viewed as a way to successfully solve both complex and simple problems. The fixation of the surrounding culture with the unacceptability of suicidal behaviors should not mislead the clinician into believing that the patient shares this view. As a class, suicidal patients generally have favorable evaluations of suicide as a way of solving problems. This tension between cultural mores and the often-anguished world of an individual who is trying to solve difficult problems is a major dynamic of the helping relationship. The most important learning point of this discussion is as follows:

- There is a paradoxical effect of suicidal behavior in that the short-term consequences are generally positive, whereas the long term consequences generate additional and more uncontrollable negative internal states and negative responses in the environment.

Instrumental Versus Expressive Functions

Another way to think about the problem-solving capacity of suicidal behavior is to see it as having both instrumental and expressive functions. The term *in-*

strumental function means using suicidal behavior with the intent of solving a problem. For example, killing oneself is an instrumental solution to the problem of suffering unbearable emotional pain. When someone is dead, there is no feeling. Being dead is an instrumental solution for the problem of feeling bad.

Expressive function means that there is a communication value to the act of attempting suicide or of talking to others about suicide. Expressive functions usually have a problem-solving overtone (e.g., an attempt to elicit help or understanding from others, to activate a social network) but can also be emotional communications in their own right. For example, suicidal patients are often very attached to black-and-white evaluations of others, themselves, and the world in which they live. This tendency toward judgmental stances leads to a variety of negative, other-directed emotions. Suicidal behavior may function to communicate anger and blame toward an offending spouse or function as a form of revenge on a sexually abusive parent. Another way to think about expressive functions is that whereas instrumental functions are self-focused, expressive functions are often other-focused.

One of the major difficulties you will encounter in working with suicidal communication is assessing the relative importance of instrumental and expressive functions for each patient. A misunderstanding can lead to negative labeling of a suicidal patient, especially one who is verbalizing intent. Terms such as "manipulative suicidal threats" may mislead the clinician into believing that a patient's suicidal verbalizations are a deliberate attempt to coerce the clinician into behaving in a certain way. In fact, the patient may be expressing, albeit unclearly, a sense of complete emotional desperation. A sound clinical framework involves assessing both the instrumental and expressive functions of suicidal behavior. If you do not have this kind of appreciation, it is likely that you and your patient may proceed on different tracks. The major clinical rule of this portion of the model is as follows:

- Suicidal behavior both can be a tool for solving particular problems and can function to communicate the patient's emotional pain and desperation.

The Basic Formula for Suicidal Crisis: The Three *Is*

How is it possible that so many people in the United States can experience a significant suicidal crisis at some point in their lives? *It is a potential experience for all of us if we experience emotional or physical pain that we believe is*

Intolerable

Inescapable

Interminable

When a person experiences emotional or physical pain that exceeds his or her threshold, the pain becomes *intolerable.* When the person believes that no strategies exist for solving the problem that is producing the pain, the pain is seen as *inescapable.* When the expectation develops that the situation that produces intense pain will not change of its own accord, the pain is viewed as *interminable.* Our position is that any person who adopts these three attitudes is likely to at least think about, if not attempt to commit, suicide.

What does it take for a person to find him- or herself in a situation that meets these criteria? There are two prototype situations. The first is an external situation that by its very nature presents the person with an overwhelming personal challenge. Examples are the sudden loss of job owing to bankruptcy of a company, the death of a spouse or child, and contracting a chronic, painful disease. Massive and unwanted social change, such as the Cultural Revolution in China in the 1970s, can present such a challenge. By most objective standards, the person is faced with overwhelmingly negative problems. The second and more pervasive type of situation occurs when the person lacks specific skills to address the demands of a situation that by itself is not overwhelming but when combined with the person's skill deficits becomes a major challenge. Examples of these types of situations might be an impending marital separation, disciplinary action on the job, chronic underemployment, and family conflict. There are two basic ways a person can exhibit dysfunction in this second type of situation:

1. The person is unwilling or unable to have the pain associated with the situation and instead of tackling the situation begins to use emotional control and avoidance strategies. With this type of dysfunction the problem remains largely unsolved.

2. The person is not using effective problem-solving tactics even though negative affect is initially being tolerated. Ineffective problem solving may result from failure to properly define the scope and nature of the problem, to select workable solutions, to follow through with problem-solving actions, or to let go of unrealistic problem-solving goals. Over time, the wear and tear of continued pain begins to produce more negative and action-oriented problem-solving behaviors, one of which is thinking about, attempting, or completing suicide.

The message is that suicidal behavior seldom occurs in a problem-solving vacuum, because it is in fact on the continuum of problem-solving options. In other words, the suicidal person truly believes that all other reasonable attempts to solve the problem have been tried and have failed. As these problem-solving options are removed from the list of possibilities, the new options become more and more extreme, particularly if a great deal of emotional pain is associated with the problem.

Clinical experience suggests that faulty problem solving evolves into suicidal behavior. Few patients with whom we have worked start out with the assumption that suicide is an effective solution; rather, they come to this belief after they have experimented with and failed with less extreme forms of problem solving. Better-functioning individuals who enter into a suicidal crisis generally have tried a variety of strategies to gain control over their moods and environmental stressors, only to see these strategies fail. These people become progressively more "locked in" on suicide as the only way out. In turn, their recognition of this fact can produce an additional fear factor that only adds to the sense of loss of emotional and behavioral control. Thinking about suicide increases the emotional burden.

In contrast, individuals who are repetitiously suicidal have come to believe that suicidal behavior is a solution for almost any problem, be it a major life stress or daily hassle. Their repeated experiments with suicidal ideation have convinced them that suicidal behavior is a strategy of first resort and is a good way to solve problems.

In both these scenarios, you are almost always treating someone who has become convinced over time that there are no other workable problem-solving options. This mind-set is a key leverage point in intervening with the suicidal patient. The focus, rather than attempting to persuade the patient that the act of suicide is intrinsically bad, is on getting the patient to discover that viable problem-solving options have been overlooked or improperly implemented. Every suicidal patient would like to find a less extreme way to solve problems but must have direct experience that the effort and patience required are worth it. This concept is often referred to as the ambivalence of the suicidal patient. The clinical theme underlying this treatment principle is as follows:

- Suicidal behavior originates under conditions of extreme emotional pain, when the person's tolerance for pain is exhausted and less extreme problem-solving strategies appear to not be working.

The Patient's Relationship to Suffering

A pivotal aspect of the suicidal crisis is the patient's relationship to his or her suffering. Our culture places a strong emphasis on feeling good, and a great variety of technology has been developed to give the appearance that people do not have to suffer. An interesting paradox arises for the person who is in emotional pain that is not likely to go away. The person struggles with the willingness to suffer. Acceptance of suffering is very, very low. When suffering occurs, the person believes that life is unfair, someone is victimizing him or her, the person lacks character or willpower, the person must deserve to suffer, and so forth. Even a person who has never been suicidal before usually undertakes an inner dialogue about the unacceptability of personal pain. In essence, the pain has to go away because the person will not accept it. This feeling causes tremendous difficulties in regulating emotional arousal, which is often experienced as being out of control. The perception of loss of emotional and behavioral control is a central feature of all suicidal crises. The person's self-evaluation processes create the conditions of low pain tolerance. As more and more provocative self-evaluations occur, acceptance is driven down and the sense of crisis increases. Chronic suicidal behavior occurs when a wider and wider range of situations tap limited problem-solving abilities in a person with an extremely low tolerance for and acceptance of any kind of suffering. This type of person suffers night and day. Although the presence of a mental disorder may introduce a new pain stimulus and impair pain tolerance, it is likely that low acceptance and pain tolerance skills are distributed normally and are just as likely to *cause* mental disorders such as depression or anxiety. This concept may explain why many patients with depression are not suicidal and many patients without depression are suicidal.

Final Comments

We believe that this learning-based, multidimensional model is a flexible tool for reframing suicidal behavior, for both clinician and patient. It objectifies the process of suicidal behavior, and it tends to reduce negative self-evaluations within the patient and pejorative labeling by the therapist. This reframing also has a strong normalizing quality; it implicitly decreases the patient's sense of social stigma and isolation. The emphasis on accepting distressing feelings while finding solutions to real-life problems is far more upbeat than focusing on what is wrong with the patient. The patient spends less time obsessing about whether he or she is crazy and more time focused on solving problems. The interventions that fall out of this approach tend to be bite-sized, concrete, and "doable" rather than global and oriented in personality change. In turn, there is a greater likelihood that the patient experiences immediate success in destabilizing the three *I*s. You should always be alert for clinical situations in which the problem-solving model is less applicable, for example, an actively psychotic patient who is hearing command hallucinations to commit suicide. However, even a severely disturbed patient at some point needs to begin solving real-life problems, which no doubt have had a bearing on the development of symptoms in the first place. As soon as a patient's cognitive abilities are capable of dealing with the rudiments of an acceptance-based problem-solving approach, it is time to use this technique.

Helpful Hints

- The essence of suicidal crisis involves the three *I*s: Emotional pain that is
  - Intolerable
  - Inescapable
  - Interminable

- Suicidal behavior is a learned, reinforced problem-solving behavior that is used when all other options seem to have failed.
- Suicidal patients as a group have a very low willingness to experience emotional pain.
- The problem-solving function of suicidal behavior is that it allows the patient to control or eliminate both internal and external problems.
- The suicidal patient views suicide as a legitimate problem-solving device, despite any social stigma attached to the behavior.

Reference

Hayes S, Strosahl K, Wilson K: Acceptance and Commitment Therapy: An Experiential Approach to Behavior Change. New York, Guilford, 1999

Selected Readings

Blumenthal SJ, Kupfer DJ: Suicide Over the Life Cycle: Risk Factors, Assessment, and Treatment of Suicidal Patients. Washington, DC, American Psychiatric Press, 1990

Linehan M: Dialectical Behavior Therapy for Borderline Personality Disorder. New York, Guilford, 1994

Maris R: Pathways to Suicide: A Survey of Self-Destructive Behaviors. Baltimore, MD, Johns Hopkins University Press, 1981

4

Assessment of Suicidal Behavior and Predisposing Factors

Blending Your Assessment With Treatment

A basic dilemma for a clinician working with a suicidal patient is the possibility that suicidal behavior will occur after the initial contact. This circumstance arises in a variety of contexts. The patient may present for help either because of intense suicidal ideation or after a suicide attempt. Alternatively, a patient may not be suicidal initially but becomes so during the course of treatment. Whatever the circumstances, you will experience pressure from a variety of sources (most external, but some internal) both to predict whether a suicide is likely to occur and, if it is, to prevent it.

There are two implicit and widely accepted assumptions that create this pressure: 1) there are specific factors that foretell suicidal behavior in a given individual (i.e., risk factors) and 2) there is a correct intervention (either medication, psychotherapy, crisis intervention, or a combination of these) that will prevent suicide from occurring. Unfortunately, very few research findings support the efficacy of these interventions. For the most part, their "validity" is an unsubstantiated part of clinical lore rather than a product of scientific research. Nevertheless, the notion that clinicians have the capability of predicting and preventing suicide has worked its way deep into the community standard of care for all the mental health disciplines. As we discuss in Chapter 3 ("A Basic Model of Suicidal Behavior"), most malpractice and negligence lawsuits hinge on the implicit truth of these assumptions. Without these assumptions, civil litigation after a suicide would become less frequent.

In this chapter we highlight the many difficulties with accurate suicide risk prediction and introduce an alternative approach in which assessment is used to reframe suicidal behavior in a way that contributes to the success of treatment. This assessment model will allow you to incorporate suicidal behavior into the fabric of treatment. It will also let you evaluate and target one or more of the many underlying conditions that may lead a patient to use suicidal behavior instead of other, more effective problem-solving methods.

Remember, assessment should not be a disconnected act. It is a part of treatment.

Prediction of Suicidal Behavior: Clinical Lore Versus Clinical Research

Clinicians are almost always under pressure to figure out whether a patient is going to attempt suicide in a very short time frame, usually no more than 24–48 hours. Few patients can sustain a bona fide suicidal crisis longer than that. The prediction question is short-term—that is, whether your patient is going to engage in suicidal behavior in the next couple of days. Most states require you to take preventive action if you determine there is an imminent risk of suicide, usually defined as the immediate and likely threat of a suicide attempt. The question then becomes how to differentiate patients who are thinking of suicide from those who will actually make an attempt. As we discuss in Chapter 2 ("The Clinician's Emotions, Values, Legal Exposure, and Ethics"), thinking about suicide is common in the general population, whereas completed suicide is rare. This disparity leads to an inherent prediction problem referred to as a *base rate problem*. The event in question that must be predicted (i.e., suicide) is so infrequent that the statistical and clinical accuracy of a prediction is nearly nonexistent. Practically speaking, it means that thinking or talking about suicide is not really an accurate predictor of attempting suicide in the next 24–48 hours. Why? Because there will be several thousand such patients for every one completed suicide. If you like playing the lottery, you will have a good understanding of these odds.

Think of the problem this way. You have had a really bad night in the emergency department and have seen 1,000 suicide attempters. A history of suicide attempts is one of the most significant risk factors for suicide. One percent, or 10, of these patients will die by suicide in the next year. You are a very good clinician and operate with 80% efficiency in this situation (most of us are not that good). You will correctly identify 8 of 10 of the individuals. However, because of the small base rate, you will have 192 (out of 990) false positives. Because of your excellent clinical skills, you have identified 200 most-at-risk individuals, 8 of whom will actually die by suicide in the next year. But you cannot be more precise than that. What will your intervention be?

Many clinicians deal with this problem by hospitalizing patients who fit a *high-risk profile*. If these factors were evenly applied throughout the United States at any given point in time, in all probability there would not be enough hospital beds in all medical and psychiatric facilities to hold the high-risk patients, especially if they were kept there for the 6 months to a year that constitutes the time frame for most risk studies. Unfortunately, many clinicians ignore this *false-positive dilemma*. They are unaware of or do not sufficiently consider the possible invasive, destructive side effects of hospitalization on a presumably high-risk patient who never would have gone on to attempt or complete suicide. The potential benefits must be weighed against the prime directive of mental health ethics: Do not harm the patient with the treatment. We discuss this issue further in Chapter 8 ("Hospitals and Suicidal Behavior: A Complex Relationship").

Risk Prediction Systems

For more than three decades, suicidologists have tried to overcome the prediction problem by developing statistically derived risk prediction systems. The strategy is to compare key environmental, personality, historical, and biological characteristics of persons who commit suicide with those of control subjects (e.g., nonsuicidal psychiatric patients). Variables that emerge as significant in these comparisons are then combined into prediction equations. The goal is to find the best set of factors that correctly identify who is likely to commit suicide. There have been many investigations of this sort, and the result has been a number of suicide risk prediction instruments. In general, these instruments provide clinical information useful in its own right, but they are fundamentally unable to do anything more than identify that a patient is in an elevated risk group for suicide. This is *not* the same as defining imminent risk.

The true test of a suicide risk prediction system is whether it can correctly identify before the fact who will commit suicide and who will attempt suicide. This ability requires prospective studies of patients at risk to see which factors actually are predictive of suicidal behavior. These studies are very expensive to conduct because they require large sample sizes (the base rate problem) and the development of sophisticated tracking procedures. Several major studies of this kind have been conducted. In two of these studies (Goldstein et al. 1991; Pokorny 1983) the investigators examined the panoply of suicide risk factors derived from the many previous studies in this area. The results of the two studies were amazingly consistent: There is almost no predictive power even when high-risk patients are followed for years. Remember, you, the clinician, are being asked not about years but about hours or days. Two studies of the Beck Hopelessness Scale (Beck et al. 1985, 1989) produced slightly more promising results. In both studies, over a multiyear follow-up period approximately 80% of eventual suicides were correctly predicted on the basis of hopelessness scores obtained at the start of inpatient or outpatient treatment. However, the time frame needed to develop this result was years from the initial contact. In a short-time-frame study (Strosahl et al. 1984) of the same instrument, we found that the Beck Hopelessness Scale misclassified 100% of high-lethality suicide attempters admitted to an inpatient psychiatric service.

What conclusions can be drawn about suicide prediction? First, it is difficult if not impossible to clinically intervene and prevent a behavior that cannot be accurately predicted. Second, previous research has not been conducted using a clinically relevant time frame; we have no way of knowing whether acute risk factors are the same as postevent factors. Third, a community standard of care is needed that does not misstate clinicians' capabilities in terms of suicide prediction and prevention. It is difficult enough to work with a suicidal patient without the added pressure of making an impossible prediction.

Assessing Suicidal Behavior

The systematic interview of a suicidal patient is most important. It will yield useful clinical information and produce a thorough and relevant clinic record. In this interview, it is necessary to remember some basic principles. First, recall that there are many forms of suicidal behavior, and the forms may vary in frequency, intensity, and duration. *Frequency* means how often specific episodes of suicidal behavior, ideation, or verbalization occur. *Intensity* is a measure of how concentrated the suicidal behavior is at any given point in time. *Duration* is how long an episode of suicidal behavior lasts. These dimensions vary independently; measurement of one cannot be taken as a measure of the others. In general, we look at increases in frequency, intensity, and duration as an indicator of severity. Patients tend to respond with the most alarm to increased intensity, followed by duration.

Second, always remember that asking a patient about suicidal behavior will not cause the patient to commit suicide. Rather than being distressed, the patient is often relieved that the question is asked. It puts an end to what often has been a carefully kept secret and a source of personal shame and humiliation. Asking once is not enough. Some individuals develop suicidal behavior during treatment. Others initially deny it. It is a good idea to include a question about suicidal behavior in each session you have, even with patients for whom this issue does not seem to be pertinent.

Third, a willingness to disclose suicidal ideation does not place the patient at less risk. Some authors of clinical reports suggest that some patients with truly lethal tendencies deny any suicidal intent, but results of systematic research have not substantiated this notion. All communication about suicidal intent is equally valid. If you detect hesitancy or another form of nonverbal communication when asking about suicide, pursue the question. Make sure your patient knows it is all right to talk about this topic. Remember, suicidal communication and ideation are features of suffering.

Fourth, suicidal ideation is not primarily an emotional feeling. It is more accurately described as a thought about how to solve a particular set of problems. Often the problem is that the patient is unwilling to experience some type of negative private event, such as depression, anxiety, anger, traumatic flashbacks, and disturbing physical sensations. As we describe in Chapter 3 ("A Basic Model of Suicidal Behavior"), suicidal thinking is really in the service of solving the problem of not wanting to feel bad. When suicidal thinking is assessed as if it were a feeling (as opposed to a response to other unacceptable experiences), there is a danger that more basic negative feelings get pushed down the priority list. Ask the patient to describe the problem that would be solved if he or she were dead. This is a better, more direct way of accessing basic negative emotional states.

Finally, be sure to collect the information that is in support of your specific clinical purpose. Going through textbook suicide risk factors for their own sake can be a futile exercise and can be antitherapeutic if the exercise leaves your patient with a sense of not being understood. Be sure to collect information that can be used in a positive set of interventions. As presented in Tables 4–1 and 4–2, it is important to differentiate what we label "background" and "foreground" data. Background data are typically historical information that cannot change because it has already developed and places the patient in a higher level of relative risk (e.g., a prior suicide attempt). Foreground factors are associated with the patient's current suicidality and with contemporary influences that might elevate the patient's reliance on suicidal behavior (e.g., current alcohol consumption). As a rule, be aware of but place less emphasis on background factors and focus on the current suicidal behavior and the factors that would drive the patient toward or deter the patient from attempting or completing suicide. Pay close attention to the patient's suicide-specific beliefs and expectancies. For example, patients who believe strongly that suicide would solve their problems with only minimal negative drawbacks are more likely to have engaged in high-intent suicide attempts. A simple scaling question asked after problems leading to suicidality have been described (On a 1–5 scale, with 1 meaning not effective at all and 5 meaning extremely effective, how effective would suicide be as a way to solve your problems?) will give you this information (Chiles et al. 1989). The other side of the equation is just as important. Strosahl et al. (1992) found that in a sample of hospitalized suicide attempters, the importance attached to survival and coping beliefs as reasons for going on with life despite current problems was a more important predictor of suicide intent than was hopelessness. When the suicide-as-problem-solving question and ratings of survival and coping atti-

Table 4–1.   Key factors in assigning risk for suicidal behavior

Risk factor	Question format
1. Positive evaluation of suicidal behavior	1. How effective would suicide be in solving your problems? On a 1–5 scale, 1 = not effective, 5 = completely effective (+ = 3 or above)
2. Low ability to tolerate emotional pain (intolerable)	2. If your current situation didn't change, could you tolerate the way you feel? On a 1–5 scale, 1 = could not tolerate at all, 5 = could tolerate it well (+ = 3 or below)
3. Hopelessness (interminable)	3A. As you look into the future, do you see things getting better in your life as a result of either your own efforts or natural change? On a 1–5 scale, 1 = nothing will change, things will stay bad, 5 = sure that the future will be better (+ = 3 or below) *or* 3B. Beck Hopelessness Scale = 8 or above
4. Inescapability	4. In your current situation, does it seem that no matter what you do, things just seem to stay bad or get worse? On a 1–5 scale, 1 = what I do has made a lot of difference, 5 = what I do has had no effect at all (+ = 3 or above)
5. Low survival and coping beliefs	5A. When you think about reasons for not killing yourself, how important are the idea that life is intrinsically worth living, curiosity about your future, and your desire to see this situation through to the end? On a 1–5 scale, 1 = these reasons are not important at all, 5 = these reasons are extremely important in my wanting to stay alive (+ = 3 or below) *or* 5B. Survival and Coping Beliefs scale average score is 3.00 or below (see Appendix C, Reasons for Living Inventory)

tudes are compared, the problem-solving question can be evaluated in a clinically richer context. This topic is discussed further in Chapters 5 through 8 ("Outpatient Interventions With Suicidal Patients," "The Repetitiously Suicidal Patient," "Managing Suicidal Emergencies," and "Hospitals and Suicidal Behavior"). Although clinicians are often told to focus on the plan-availability-lethality triangle (Do you have a plan? Do you have a method? Is the means to enact your method readily available? How lethal is the plan?),

Table 4–2.   Foreground and background assessment points with the suicidal patient

Background	Finding	Foreground	Finding
1. Prior suicide attempt	Present	1A. Current suicidal ideation	Present
		a. Frequency of episodes	Daily increasing
		b. Intensity of thoughts	Detailed images, trouble fighting them off
		c. Duration of episodes	At least 30 minutes, increasing in length
		and/or	
		1B. Beck Scale for Suicide Ideation (BSS) score ≥18	
2. Suicide intent in prior acts	Present	2. Preparatory behavior	Present
a. Expectation about lethality	Believed death was likely	a. Security means	Means are available
		b. Honor code	Suicide attempts made, others promised
b. Attempts to avoid detection	Strong, discovery was a fluke	c. Attempts to elude	Others have been misled about whereabouts, behavior is planned in a social vacuum
c. Final arrangements	Made	d. Final arrangements	New will written, belongings given away, suicide note written
		e. Time frame is established	Date is set, "anniversary of another suicide"

Table 4–2. Foreground and background assessment points with the suicidal patient (*continued*)

Background	Finding	Foreground	Finding
3. Medical lethality of prior acts		3. Current drug or alcohol abuse	Present; increasing consumption
a. Type of method	Very lethal		
b. Condition upon discovery	Unconscious/semiconscious		
c. Medical condition	Required real emergency department/intensive care unit services		
4. Family history of suicide	Present in first-degree family member	4. Current psychiatric condition	Depressive disorder, schizoaffective disorder, substance abuse disorder
		5. Current physical health	Poor; chronic disease or pain
		6. Current negative life stress	High; major financial, job, or relationship problems or loss
		7. Current social support	Low; social alienation or only negative supports available

experience suggests that shifting the focus to suicide-specific beliefs and positive life-sustaining beliefs allows for a much more upbeat problem-solving intervention.

Using Assessment to Reframe Suicidal Behavior

For many clinicians, there is the assessment phase of treatment and then there is the treatment phase of treatment. When the clinician is in the suicide assessment mode, there can often be little room for positive movement because the focus is on preventing something negative. Conversely, clinicians can have great difficulty when they are in the treatment mode and are interrupted by a distraught patient in a suicidal crisis requiring assessment activity. This distinction comes from the traditional medical model, which requires that a formal operating diagnosis be made before appropriate treatment can begin. But does the traditional model work in the care of suicidal patients? Certainly this approach is necessary when major mental illness is present and appropriate medication selection is needed. However, most suicidal patients need both a diagnostic assessment and an intervention that starts at first contact. For this reason, you should use the assessment process as part of, rather than distinct from, treatment proper.

Take, for example, the initial interview with a suicidal patient. In the following two vignettes, we demonstrate prevention-focused assessment and treatment-focused assessment. While reading them, think carefully about the emotional tone created in each sequence.

Prevention-Focused Assessment

> Therapist: I understand from what you're telling me that you're under a lot of stress on the job and your marriage isn't going well either. You're obviously pretty depressed.... Have you been thinking about suicide?
>
> Patient: Well, I've had some thoughts like that.
>
> Therapist: Can you tell me how seriously you're thinking about it?... By that I mean do you have a specific way that you would do it?... Do you think about it pretty much daily?
>
> Patient: I've been thinking about it quite a bit lately but I'm not sure I'd actually do it.
>
> Therapist: Do you have a method or plan about what you would do?

Patient: I usually imagine driving my car through a curve up in the mountains.

Therapist: Have you actually driven your car around that curve and imagined that you went straight?

Patient: Yes, I drive that road quite a bit as part of my job, and, sometimes, I imagine that I just end it all. That way, my wife and kids would get my life insurance. At least that way, they'd have something positive to remember me by.

Therapist: So you've been having these thoughts more often lately, is that right?

Patient: Yes, but it's not something I think about all the time; just when I'm having a lousy day. I have had quite a few lousy days lately.

Therapist: Well, I'm hearing some things that make me concerned that you might actually try to kill yourself if you had a real bad day. I'm wondering.... Would you be willing to make an agreement with me that you will not try anything like that without first calling me to talk about it? I'd like us to agree that you won't try anything like this for the time being while we work on your problems.

Patient: I suppose I can agree to that.

Treatment-Focused Assessment

Therapist: You've told me that you've got some pretty big problems in your life right now, including problems with your job and your marriage. Sometimes when people feel like there are no solutions to problems like these, they begin to think about suicide as one way to take care of the problem. Have you thought about suicide as one way of solving these problems?

Patient: Well, I've had some thoughts like that recently.

Therapist: When you think about suicide as an option here, what specific aspects of the problem do you think would be solved if you killed yourself?

Patient: Well, I wouldn't have to go work and deal with my crummy supervisor; if I were dead, then my wife and I certainly couldn't argue as much as we have.

Therapist: So, the thing that you imagine being better if you committed suicide is that you wouldn't have to participate in these conflicts, for example, with your boss or with your wife. Another way of saying this is that suicide might help you with the problem of feeling bad as a result of these interactions. Suicidal thinking or behavior serves the purpose of helping you gain control over these unwanted feelings. Does that make sense?

Patient: Yeah, I suppose I've just about had it with feeling frustrated and angry all the time, and very little I've tried gets rid of it. As many times
as I've tried to approach the situation more positively, I'm just getting
to believe that nothing is really going to make a difference.

Therapist: So, in addition to feeling bad, frustrated, and angry about what
these interactions do to you, you're also getting pessimistic that anything you do to solve the problems is going to work, is that right? It
sounds like the more you try to ratchet down on these painful feelings,
the stronger they get. As they get stronger, you get more desperate in
your search for some way to control them. Suicide might be one tactic
that would help you gain that kind of control.

Patient: Yeah, I guess it is my last resort, and I feel like I'm getting to that
point now.

Therapist: Before you get to that point, would it make sense for us to work
together to explore what you've actually done to try to solve the problem of feeling you have no emotional control and to see if we can come
up with something that might work better and doesn't involve you
having to be dead?

Patient: I suppose I can agree to that.

These two vignettes show a contrasting style of approaching the patient's
suicidality. Table 4–3 summarizes contrasting strategies generated by the as-
sessment-only versus the assessment/treatment-oriented model. In the more
assessment-focused vignette, the therapist is most interested in collecting data
about the suicidal behavior per se and trying to determine risk. The implicit
focus of the interview is to prevent the occurrence of suicide by examining the
patient's intent. In this approach, very few concepts that are integral to problem-solving treatment have been used. In a sense, the issue of suicide is on
center stage and is the *problem* that the therapist is going to focus on.

Conversely, a therapist using the treatment-focused approach is more
likely to validate and understand the patient's suicidal ideation and increasing
suicidal intent. Moreover, the issue is reframed in the context of emotional
control and avoidance and problem-solving behavior. The effect is to legiti-
mize the occurrence of suicidal ideation as a response to developing pessimism, frustration, and anger while keeping the door open that other solutions
might be available. Although the therapist is asking the patient to defer the
decision to commit suicide until other problem-solving options have been examined, this step certainly is not the primary clinical intervention. The therapist has gleaned much information about the patient's affective state and the

Table 4–3. Comparison of assessment/risk-oriented versus assessment/treatment-oriented approaches to the suicidal patient

Clinical issue	Assessment/risk oriented	Assessment/treatment oriented
1. Focus of session	Assess and manage suicide risk	Reframe suicidality as problem solving
2. Importance of knowing suicide risk factors	Very important, central part of interaction	Less important, collected in problem-solving context
3. Importance of assigning "reliable risk"	Central to type and frequency of treatment	Less important, suicide potential is not predictable
4. Risk management concerns	Very high, focus on risk factors, be prepared to take strong steps to protect patient	Low, suicidal behavior per se cannot be prevented; focus on patient's underlying problems
5. Stance regarding ongoing suicidal behavior	Prohibitive, requires ongoing detection and prevention	Anticipated, forms a basis for collecting data about problem solving
6. Legitimacy of suicidal behavior	It is the problem; the goal is to get rid of it	It is a legitimate but costly form of problem solving
7. Time allotment for discussing suicidality	Much more session time	Much less session time
8. Prevention orientation	Most strategies built around preventing suicidal behavior	Fewer prevention strategies

patient's willingness to accept negative emotions and general problem-solving style by *not focusing* on the issue of suicidal behavior. When a patient is acutely suicidal, approaching the problem from this angle immediately reassures the patient. This approach not only validates what the patient believes is an abnormal, stigmatized event (i.e., thinking seriously about suicide) but also begins to create some perspective on how people come to consider suicide an option. Although the therapist is still able to gather relevant information about the patient's suicidal intent, the general flow of the session is much calmer and more accepting of the patient's suffering and frustration.

Whenever possible, you should attempt to use acceptance-based problem-solving reframing when discussing suicidal ideation or suicide intent. *Ideation* refers to the act of thinking about suicide, whereas *intent* represents the patient's developing commitment to engage in some sort of overt behavior. It is important to understand that the movement from ideation to intent is probably based on certain types of cognitive appraisals of suicide as a useful problem-solving device. Thus problem-solving language blended with a recasting of the patient's basic agenda (to eliminate unacceptable feeling states) is enormously powerful in that it links the patient's prior experience of low-intent ideation with current higher intent as a form of problem solving. The shift from mild ideation to serious intent is scary for the patient and is often interpreted as evidence of being out of control. When you are able to explain this type of experience in a simple yet credible model, basic features of an acute suicidal crisis are being addressed even while the assessment is being conducted. If you can at the same time validate and normalize intense suicidal ideation while shifting the focus to problem solving and tolerance of emotional pain, there will often be an immediate reduction in suicidal intent and ideation.

Using Self-Monitoring to Study Suicidal Behavior

In keeping with the principle that assessment and treatment should be used interchangeably with the suicidal patient, it is important to find ways to incorporate assessment strategies into ongoing treatment. One of the most effective strategies is to use self-monitoring assignments between treatment sessions. Self-monitoring is a flexible and powerful therapeutic tool, and its reactive treatment effects have been well documented with a variety of clinical problems. Reactive treatment effects occur when the act of collecting the information has an impact on the behavior that is being studied. When a suicidal patient collects information about episodes of suicidal ideation, there is a corresponding shift from a participant mentality to an observer mentality. This cognitive shift is fundamental to many behavior change processes. It is much easier to see what needs to be done from the viewpoint of an observer than it is from the viewpoint of the participant. Suicidal ideation always looks and feels different when it is being studied as opposed to when it is being experienced.

The self-monitoring strategy also tends to bring ongoing (and often undisclosed) suicidal ideation or behavior into the mainstream of therapy. For example, if a patient experiences suicidal ideation as treatment continues, a self-monitoring assignment can be agreed to that will be used to attempt to identify environmental triggers for suicidal thinking. Along with these triggers, ask the patient to list the associated thoughts and feelings. The patient may keep a daily log of intensity, frequency, and duration of suicidal episodes or may carefully track the time of day when suicidal ideation tends to occur. These tasks are examples of using what the patient brings into therapy to promote an aboveboard approach to suicidality while remaining committed to finding solutions to the patient's real-life dilemmas.

Prescribing Self-Monitoring Tasks

Often the patient feels that resisting thinking about suicide by using sheer willpower is the only way to get better. Paradoxically, for many, the more suicidal ideation is resisted, the worse it tends to become. To most patients this paradox is the epitome of being out of control. The patient decides to stop thinking about suicide yet ironically finds the suicidal ideation getting bigger and stronger each day. Prescriptive self-monitoring tasks can reverse this misguided notion about therapeutic change by providing a scientific paradigm in which to study the suicidal behavior rather than resist it. There are times when the patient is so locked-in on the willpower strategy that self-monitoring can be used in an almost paradoxical way. You can provide an eloquent rationale for the need to study suicidal impulses so patients can learn more about their topography. You can predict that it will be very difficult for the patient to make the kinds of changes that would be required to problem solve events in a nonsuicidal way without allowing suicidal options to exist. Using a self-monitoring framework, you can distract the patient from the futile task of resisting repetitive and self-reinforcing cognitive processes, knowing that the patient's negative attention in fact acts as a reinforcement for the recurrence of suicidal ideation. Instead, your patient has permission to have the suicidal ideation and record it for further analysis. This approach communicates your confidence in the patient's capacity to have and at the same time think about suicidal impulses. This type of intervention is usually effective with patients who are locked-in on the strategy of using willpower to get rid of suicidal ideation. It is intended to reduce your patient's level of discomfort about the out-of-control experience of failing at the willpower game.

Collaboration in Data Collection

It is important to develop assignments in collaboration with your patient. Collaboration makes the activity relevant to your patient's problems and leads to a greater likelihood that the patient will follow through with the assignment. It is important to include your patient in the design of self-monitoring strategies and in any written forms used to keep daily data. The therapist's eye is always on making the process user-friendly and focusing on issues that are important to the patient. When a self-monitoring assignment has been generated, you should make sure the patient feels the assignment is possible, given all of the emotional twists and turns in the patient's environment. Your patient should feel ownership of the self-monitoring assignment and the way in which data are eventually used. This aspect of the process increases the patient's commitment to developing the observer-scientist perspective on the problem and yields much greater compliance rates. The therapist who hands the patient a piece of paper and says, "Here, keep this information for me. It is important," is inviting failure.

It is also important to see such homework activities as an integral part of the intervention structure. These activities are not something that should be tacked on in the last 2 minutes of an interaction with a patient but should be the focus of good, solid collaborative work. When your patient agrees to put in the time and effort to collect information, you cannot ignore or forget about this assignment in the next session, as happens with distressing frequency when homework assignments are simply tacked on. If a patient takes the time and effort to produce the information and then is ignored by the therapist in the next session, between-session activity will quickly disappear. The patient has just learned to do less work between sessions.

You should devote the first part of each session to thoroughly reviewing any homework assignments that have been developed with the patient in previous sessions. You should use the information in a way that tells the patient it is linked to the eventual success of therapy. Your patient should be actively involved in the process of looking for trends and for important comparison points. It is useful to start the review process by asking the patient to discuss any possible trends in the information collected since the last session. When a dialogue develops around the patient's perspective on the data, the process is much more likely to lead to important discoveries by the patient.

Using Self-Report Inventories

As mentioned earlier in "Risk Prediction Systems," many suicide-risk instruments are of limited predictive value to the clinician. There are, however, occasions when self-report inventories and scaling questions are useful in the process of assessment and treatment. For example, when the patient has a mental condition such as depressive or anxiety disorder that is related to the suicidal preoccupations, it makes sense to periodically administer depression or anxiety inventories to monitor mood levels. A therapist interested in suicide-specific thoughts can use the Beck Hopelessness Scale (Beck et al. 1985), the Reasons for Living Inventory (Appendix C), or scaling questions about problem solving and tolerance for emotional distress. In general, self-report assessment processes inform the clinician of the patient's current emotional state and can suggest useful therapeutic targets. These assessments also can be used to classify a patient according to a comparison population at risk of suicidal behavior. If a patient reports high levels of hopelessness with low importance attached to reasons for living and a positive evaluation of suicide as a problem-solving option, that patient likely has a strong commitment to suicidal behavior. If the patient has been slow to divulge this information, a self-report assessment process can be a lead-in for you to ask the patient directly about the presence of suicidal thinking. Occasionally, you will also want to look at various characteristics of the patient's suicidal behavior repertoire. Toward this end, the Suicidal Thinking and Behaviors Questionnaire (Appendix D) is a very useful summary measure. Also recommended for the assessment of contemporary suicidal ideation is the Beck Scale for Suicide Ideation (Beck et al. 1979), an interview-based measure of the intensity of suicidal thinking. The most important principle is to use assessment devices when they fit a particular purpose relevant to treatment. An example may be to provide a profile of the patient at the outset of therapy or to use it for some other specific purpose after therapy has begun. For instance, you may be interested in the amount of change a patient has undergone over the course of several sessions. In this case, it is wise to administer and re-administer these questionnaires.

The principal benefit of using self-report inventories is that they provide a quantifiable way of comparing the patient with various clinical populations who have various clinical syndromes. Interestingly, patients often feel more positive about the therapist when inventories are used at the outset of therapy. Using inventories often creates the impression that the therapy is credible and that the practitioner is very knowledgeable. For the patient who is scared and out of control, it is reassuring to encounter an interviewer who seems to have special knowledge and who seems to have a systematic plan for bringing order out of chaos.

Assessing Predisposing Factors

Now that you are familiar with the basic model of suicidal behavior and are equipped to directly assess various aspects of suicidal behavior, you can begin to assess for characteristics that you will want to tackle in the treatment of your patient. Recall that suicidal behavior is the end result of a variety of skill and attitudinal variables that combine to make suicidal behavior an option for the patient. Numerous empirical studies have been conducted to examine various personality, environmental, and interpersonal characteristics of suicidal patients. Unfortunately, most of these studies were conducted with patients who think about or verbalize suicidal intent or attempt suicide. The extent to which these characteristics can be generalized to patients who commit suicide is very much in debate. For this reason, as we go over these characteristics and help you assess them as part of your clinical workup, you should remember our message in the previous section ("Using Self-Report Inventories"): There is no scientific evidence that indicates a clinician armed with the results of assessments or any other pieces of client information can accurately predict a suicide or suicide attempt. To help make sense of the vast array of information in this area, we highlight some of the core research findings and then describe how certain of these characteristics will manifest themselves in your office. Finally, we introduce you to an easy-to-use assessment device that will allow you to profile where each of your patients stands on these various dimensions (see Table 4–4, later in this section).

Thinking Style

The most widely cited personality feature of suicidal patients is cognitive rigidity. Suicidal patients have trouble being flexible. They become stuck on one and only one version of the problem. Perspective taking is extremely difficult. In a sense, the patient cannot back away from life problems long enough to get any fresh ideas. There is an overreliance on passive problem-solving strategies, which rely on luck, spontaneous change, or the actions of others. This overreliance leads to the well-known phenomenon of tunnel vision, which refers to the marked narrowing of the person's problem-solving field. Problems are defined in rigid, value-laden terms. This manner of thinking tends to spawn black-and-white value judgments about what the person ought to do.

Effective problem solving requires a specific set of skills. Suicidal people often have less of these abilities. It is not clear whether this phenomenon is a state or a trait. Suicidal crises may induce these characteristics, or they may already exist in individuals who are prone to suicidal behavior. In any event, the suicidal person generates few alternative solutions to a particular situation, prematurely rejects effective solutions as having been tried and failed, and looks for solutions with positive short-term consequences without much consideration of long-term effects. There is a preference for passive or avoidance-based solutions (e.g., quit a job rather than confront a supervisor).

This problem-solving style leads the suicidal person to regard suicidal behavior as an effective problem-solving device. It precludes having to rely on and influence people in the external world and instead brings control over the solution entirely within the individual. Although it may be argued that suicide is an active form of problem solving, we regard this attitude as the quintessence of passive responding. A common feature of the clinical dialogue with a suicidal patient is the issue of short-term versus long-term consequences. The suicidal patient is interested in short-term fixes and is less than receptive to discussions about the long-term implications of his or her behavior. For example, trying to persuade a patient that a failed suicide attempt will probably result in more problems in the long term is generally a futile therapeutic exercise.

Tolerance for Negative Feelings

Two characteristics of emotional functioning tend to exacerbate suicidal crises. The first is the lack of effective techniques for regulating emotional arousal. The suicidal person has no way of turning off the physiological pump that provides the physical platform for chronic emotional overarousal. A common clinical complaint is emotional exhaustion or numbness related to prolonged exposure to excessive physiological arousal. Developing behaviors that serve to relax the patient physically or to offset "ratcheting" cognitions is very important in working through a suicidal crisis. The suicidal patient experiences intense and variable mood states that can change very rapidly with or without an apparent cause. Often the patient will complain that feeling bad is hard to accept but is not as bad as the sense of being out of control physically and emotionally.

The second clinical feature in this area is a low willingness to accept negative private experiences, whether they be emotions, thoughts, memories, or bodily sensations. It is not unusual for suicidal patients to say things like "I can't stand this feeling of anxiety" or "No matter what I do, I end up feeling guilty." It is as if the only goal of being alive is to somehow conquer any negative personal material that shows up in the patient's life. As a consequence, impulsive problem solving emerges as a more and more favored type of solution. Intense and prolonged negative affect leads the person to make desperation-driven decisions. We believe this attitude also explains why addictive behaviors such as drinking, bulimia, and drug use have been shown to co-occur with suicidal behavior. In the attempt to avoid feeling bad, the person can and will select any number of poisons, including deadly ones. In the end, all of these escape and avoidance behaviors are birds of a feather.

Social Behavior

In general, a suicidal person is not interpersonally effective, although it is not clear whether this condition is a cause or a result of suicidal behavior patterns.

Research suggests that suicidal persons experience elevated levels of social anxiety, fear of rejection, and chronic feelings of inferiority. Suicidal patients are usually socially isolated and may have few people who can offer social support. Relationships are often marked by excessive dependency, submissiveness, and avoidance of interpersonal conflict. The suicidal person generally places a premium on maintaining the appearance of normalcy around others. This facade can be misleading to the therapist, who may overestimate the patient's social and behavioral competence. The artificial social competence usually deteriorates when the patient has to address the daily requirements of actively participating in relationships.

Social supports are usually limited both in terms of numbers of potentially helpful persons and in the usefulness of the support provided. Principal figures in the support system may be equivocal in their support of the patient. This situation is particularly true with family members who may at the same time be hopeful that the patient will solve problems and be angry that the difficulties existed in the first place.

We use the term *competent social support* as a constant reminder that some individuals in the patient's social support network are actually the opposite of supportive. In assessing the patient's social support network, it is important that you identify the real versus the imagined social support structure. Many a therapeutic plan has failed when the patient accesses a social support only to be barraged with criticism, moralizing, and useless directives. In other situations involving patients with chronic suicidal behavior patterns, the patient's "friend" may be a fellow suicidal patient that your patient met during his or her most recent hospitalization. One of us (K.S.) set up a social support plan involving an intimate other of an acutely suicidal patient, believing that the patient's partner would be a source of reassurance and positive direction. Over time, as the social support plan consistently failed to help reduce the patient's suicidality, it was discovered that the chief content of social support interactions during suicidal crises was to develop a joint suicide pact.

Behavior Change Skills

Suicidal individuals are poor at applying self-control skills or personal behavior modification strategies. The suicidal person is often somewhat of a perfectionist and may liberally use punishment and withdrawal of rewards as a means of coercing "better" behavior. Because of the anxiety generated by this self-reinforcement style, the suicidal patient often reports a long history of failed attempts at behavior change. Because the internal self-reward system is dysfunctional, the patient drifts to external reinforcements such as alcohol and drugs because of the intrinsically rewarding properties of these substances. Therapeutic interventions that rely exclusively on self-reinforcement strategies (such as willpower) often do not work. Admonitions to immediately change behavior (If you are going to be in therapy with me, you have to stop your suicidal behavior!) are meaningless because the person usually has negative experiences with willpower cures. The "all you need to do" admonitions, whether from you, a family member, or a friend, can be quite disheartening. Advice such as "Just be nicer to your spouse" or "Quit worrying about your health" is rarely useful. If the patient were able to generate such behavior change on the basis of simple insights, it is highly unlikely the patient would be a patient in the first place.

Life Stress

Life stress has long been associated with suicidal behavior and is an important way of gauging the degree of disturbance in the patient's environment. Stresses frequently are chronic (e.g., sustained unemployment, inadequate social network), and suicidal patients have a much higher than normal rate of acute stresses (e.g., separation or divorce, recent death of loved one). Daily hassles to which the person is continually exposed wear down emotional resistance and probably create a basic predisposition to suicidal crisis when a truly negative life event occurs. A commonly reported problem in working with suicidal patients, especially repetitious patients, is the crisis-of-the-week syndrome. In essence, the patient presents with a new life stress at each therapy session, making it difficult if not impossible for the therapist to implement a basic treatment plan. This problem suggests there are strong benefits to developing a focus on handling routine matters in one's daily life rather than simply solving big problems. Indeed, the learning model emphasizes that small solutions multiplied over time are the way that the patient can turn his or her life around. Particularly with patients enduring chronic environmental stresses, the notion of heroic change is just as destructive as that of willpower cures. Patients rarely get into such situations overnight, and the way out is likely to require small steps.

Predisposing Factors Assessment Tool

Table 4–4 a clinical protocol for profiling the condition of your patient with respect to the major predisposing factors. This tool allows you to characterize your patient at the point of entry into treatment and can function as a clinical outcome measure. Remember that the presence of many predisposing factors does not mean your patient is at imminent risk of suicide. This tool is designed to help you locate the treatment targets (i.e., skill deficits) that you will attempt to address in your treatment. The patient's suicidality is a by-product of these more basic underlying deficits. We strongly encourage you not only to profile your patient's suicidal action tendencies (background and foreground relative risk) but also to immediately assess skill deficits the patient is presenting that will become the focus of your therapeutic interventions.

Table 4–4. Personality and environmental factor assessment for suicidal patients

Cognitive style (1–5 rating[a])
1. Black-or-white, judgmental thinking (heavily into right and wrong, good and bad)
2. Rigid, inflexible cognitive style (things just are the way they are)

Problem-solving style (1–5 rating[a])
1. Thinks about short-term rather than long-term effects of actions
2. Has positive expectancies regarding suicide as a problem-solving strategy
3. Lacks confidence in insight; actions speak louder than words
4. Poor problem-solving skills
   - Has trouble identifying problems and their sources
   - Generates fewer possible solutions
   - Prematurely rejects potentially viable alternatives
   - Exhibits passive problem-solving behaviors
   - Poorly executes problem-solving strategies

Emotional pain and suffering (1–5 rating[a])
1. Tendency toward chronic feelings of anger, guilt, depression, anxiety, and boredom
2. Significant source of external distress (e.g., interpersonal loss or death)
3. Intense, unstable affect with rapid changes in nature of feelings

Emotionally avoidant coping style
1. Difficulty tolerating negative affect; cannot regulate arousal once it starts
2. Belief that painful feelings are wrong or toxic or are evidence of weak character or failure in living

Table 4–4.   Personality and environmental factor assessment for suicidal patients *(continued)*

3. Impulsive attempts to eliminate affect (e.g., cutting, drinking, drug taking, or binge eating)

Interpersonal deficits

1. Lowered assertiveness, especially when alcohol problems are not present
2. Confusion of assertion and aggression when alcohol problems are present
3. Frequent severe social anxiety, often accompanied by a feeling of being "evaluated"
4. Tendency toward social isolation, dependency conflicts, or severe mistrust
5. Relationships characterized by excessive conflict and frequent "ups and downs"

Self-control deficits

1. Use of self-punishment and criticism as primary means of modifying behavior
2. Limited success with self-initiated behavior change
3. Difficulties setting small, positive goals (wants heroic solutions)

Environmental stress and social support buffers

1. Stress related to acute life stresses (e.g., job loss or separation or divorce)
2. Ongoing level of daily stress is elevated (i.e., "daily hassles")
3. Very few competent social supports to buffer stress
    * Significant others may be antagonistic to patient
    * Significant others may be poor role models for problem solving
    * Significant others may lecture, moralize, or cajole the patient
    * Significant others may offer poor advice (e.g., willpower cure)

[a]Global rating: 1 = low clinical risk; 5 = high clinical risk.

Helpful Hints

* It is almost impossible in the short term to predict who will commit suicide and who will not.
* Suicide risk prediction scales may provide useful clinical information but are not able to predict who will commit suicide or make a suicide attempt.
* There are different forms of suicidal behavior, and each can vary with respect to frequency of occurrence, duration, and intensity.
* The patient's evaluation of suicide as a problem-solving method is strongly related to ongoing suicidal behavior.
* Reframe suicidal behavior as problem-solving behavior in the service of eliminating or controlling negative private events. Asking a limited

number of questions about the patient's belief in the effectiveness of suicidal behavior as a problem-solving tactic, and the patient's willingness to "stand" negative feelings (Table 4–1) will help you assess the patient's basic stance on suicidal behavior.

- Do not differentiate between assessment and treatment with the suicidal patient; use the two strategies interchangeably.
- Differentiate background and foreground suicidal risk factors in your assessment, placing more emphasis on the foreground.
- Use instruments such as the Suicidal Thinking and Behaviors Questionnaire (Appendix D) and the Reasons for Living Inventory (Appendix C) to help quantify your assessment of both negative and positive patient factors.
- Use self-monitoring (diary keeping) homework assignments to help the patient objectify suicidal behavior.
- Be sure to involve (collaborate with) the patient in developing relevant assessment strategies.
- Always include in your initial assessment an inventory of factors predisposing individuals to suicidal behavior (Table 4–4). Predisposing factors include

    - Cognitive rigidity and poor personal problem-solving skills
    - Inability to regulate the physical and cognitive components of stress
    - Unwillingness to accept negative emotional states, cognitions, memories, or physical symptoms
    - Poor general social skills and a dearth of effective social support buffers
    - Heightened chronic and acute life stresses, including a crisis-of-the-week mentality in some patients

References

Beck A, Rush J, Shaw D, et al: Cognitive Therapy for Depression: A Treatment Manual. New York, Guilford, 1979

Beck A, Steer RA, Kovacs M, et al: Hopelessness and eventual suicide: a 10-year prospective study of patients hospitalized with suicidal ideation. Am J Psychiatry 142:559–563, 1985

Beck A, Brown G, Steer R: Prediction of eventual suicide in psychiatric inpatients by clinical ratings of hopelessness. J Consult Clin Psychol 57:309–310, 1989

Chiles JA, Strosahl KD, Ping ZY, et al: Depression, hopelessness, and suicidal behavior in Chinese and American psychiatric patients. Am J Psychiatry 146:339–344, 1989

Goldstein RB, Black DW, Nasrallah A, et al: The prediction of suicide. Arch Gen Psychiatry 48:418–422, 1991

Pokorny AD: Prediction of suicide in psychiatric patients: report of a prospective study. Arch Gen Psychiatry 40:249–257, 1983

Strosahl K, Linehan M, Chiles J: Will the real social desirability please stand up? hopelessness, depression, social desirability and the prediction of suicidal behavior. J Consult Clin Psychol 52:449–457, 1984

Strosahl K, Chiles JA, Linehan M: Prediction of suicide intent in hospitalized parasuicides: reasons for living, hopelessness and depression. Compr Psychiatry 33:366–373, 1992

Selected Readings

Beck A, Schuyler D, Herman I: Development of suicidal intent scales, in The Prediction of Suicide. Edited by Beck AT, Resnik HL, Lettieri DJ. Bowie, MD, Charles Press, 1974, pp 45–56

Beck A, Weissman A, Lester D, et al: The measurement of pessimism: the Hopelessness Scale. J Consult Clin Psychol 42:861–865, 1974

Harris EC, Barraclough BM: Suicide as an outcome for mental disorders: a meta-analysis. Br J Psychiatry 170:205–228, 1997

Linehan M, Goodstein J, Nielson S, et al: Reasons for staying alive when you're thinking of killing yourself: the Reasons for Living Inventory. J Consult Clin Psychol 51:276–286, 1983

Litman R: Predicting and preventing hospital and clinic suicides. Suicide Life Threat Behav 21:56–73, 1991

Patsiokas A, Clum G, Luscomb R: Cognitive characteristics of suicide attempters. J Consult Clin Psychol 47:478–484, 1979

Schotte DE, Clum GA: Problem-solving skills in suicidal psychiatric patients. J Consult Clin Psychol 55:49–54, 1987

5

Outpatient Interventions
With Suicidal Patients

In this chapter, we present interventions that you can use with the suicidal outpatient in a range of clinical encounters. These interventions vary from the one-time crisis session at which the goal is to stabilize the crisis and refer the patient for further treatment to techniques for establishing a longer-term treatment relationship. Regardless of the length of your involvement, the chief clinical goals and associated strategies for meeting those goals are the same: First, establish a consistent, caring, and credible therapeutic framework that will reassure your patient, and second, abate the suicidal crisis. It is critical that you understand any of your own issues, your "hot buttons," that might confound or undermine these objectives. Review Chapter 2 ("The Clinician's Emotions, Values, Legal Exposure, and Ethics") before proceeding with interventions. The attitude and behavior of the provider are often the most important determinants of successful treatment. The issue of suicidal behavior is so volatile for some clinicians that it is better for them to stabilize the immediate situation and refer a patient to another provider. Know your tolerances and what you can and cannot deal with in this area. *Knowing your limits is an important part of your competence, not a sign of personal weakness.*

An Overview of Treatment Philosophies

A suicidal crisis is a method your patient uses to confront a painful situation that he or she believes to be *inescapable, intolerable,* and *interminable*—the three *I*s. The goal of your treatment is to change one or more of these *I*s. This mission is accomplished by guiding your patient through experimental, experience-based learning. You have to show the patient that problems that are viewed as inescapable can be dealt with effectively and sometimes resolved. You have to show that negative feelings vary constantly and are responsive to change in the patient's behavior. You have to show that negative feelings can be tolerated and behavior can still be adaptive. When any or all of these three goals are even partially obtained, your patient's own competencies and resources have the opportunity to take over and complete the work.

In this chapter we show you a variety of clinical interventions focused on learning problem-solving and emotional-acceptance skills, skills that will help your patient achieve these objectives. Table 5–1 lists the basic principles of treatment.

Your patient will need to develop three skill sets. First, your patient must either learn to use existing problem-solving abilities more effectively or learn new problem-solving techniques. Developing effective problem solving addresses the notion of inescapability by enabling your patient to solve "unsolvable" problems. Second, your patient needs to develop self-awareness/self-observation strategies to observe natural and spontaneous fluctuations in emotional pain levels and to make associations between doing things a little differently and feeling better. Once made, these associations will undermine the belief that emotional pain will stay intense and unwavering and will last forever. Third, your patient needs to learn to tolerate negative feelings when they do arise through the acquisition of distancing and distraction skills. This effort will help your patient understand that although it is part of life, emotional pain does not have to be experienced as acute and overwhelming.

It is necessary to integrate the three skill sets in a manner that allows the patient to use them to address all sorts of difficulties. Although one objective of therapy is to reduce suicidal behavior, the process involves helping an individual see how *self-observation, problem solving,* and *emotional pain tolerance* are a part of building a quality life. The success of treatment is measured by the capacity to weave these three abilities into the fabric of the patient's life.

Table 5–1.   Basic principles of outpatient treatment with the suicidal patient

1. Suicidal behavior is an attempt to solve problems that are viewed as...
    *   Inescapable: You have to show that the problems can be solved.
    *   Interminable: You have to show that the negative feelings will end.
    *   Intolerable: You have to show the person that he or she can stand negative feelings.
2. Suicidal behavior is usually not effective at solving problems. It generally increases the problems or brings about new ones.
    *   Stress that suicide is a permanent solution to what is most often a temporary problem.
3. Feeling suicidal is a valid, understandable response to emotional pain.
    *   Demonstrate that you have an empathetic understanding of your patient's pain.
4. Establish the fact that it is acceptable to talk openly and honestly about suicide.
    *   Be matter of fact.
    *   Consistently assess for suicidal ideation and self-injurious behavior.
    *   Avoid value judgments about the act of suicide as cowardly, sinful, or vengeful.
5. Take a collaborative rather than a confrontational approach to the issue of suicidal behavior.
    *   Beware of power struggles over the occurrence of suicidal behavior.
    *   Offer assistance on how to solve the problem, but beware of willpower-type advice.
6. Offer attention and caring that are not contingent on suicidal behavior.
    *   Make random support phone calls.
    *   Make positive behavior assignments.
7. When possible, identify specific skill deficits that can be corrected in structured behavioral training.
    *   Interpersonal skills
    *   Stress management skills
    *   Problem-solving skills
    *   Self-control skills

In other words, do not make a distinction between the patient's journey through life and the patient's particular problem. The two are intertwined, and solutions for one are very likely solutions for the other.

Reconciling Opposites:
A Key to Managing Suicidal Behavior

The concept of reconciling opposites is critical for both understanding and working with suicidal patients. At heart, the suicidal patient is a black-and-white thinker who often struggles with conflicting beliefs about the same issue. For example, happiness and sadness are opposites; the patient views one as good, the other as bad. However, neither emotion can exist in a meaningful way without the other. Reconciling the necessity of having both happiness and sadness in one's life lends full meaning to the actual experiences of happiness and sadness. Although this concept is not new, most modern-day therapies do not work specifically at reconciling opposites and could be better characterized as linear. These therapies emphasize the role of logic and deductive reasoning as a way to run one's life. In a linear approach, if the therapist can show that the advantages of suicide do not outweigh the disadvantages, the patient is expected to be rational and stop the suicidal behavior. If the patient does not go along with this approach, the therapist might express frustration with the failing treatment process by attaching to the patient labels such as "resistant," "oppositional," and "manipulative." When the patient perceives that this labeling is occurring, a natural defensiveness can emerge that can create polarization and an adversarial relationship.

The process of reconciliation involves learning to honor and value polarities rather than feeling that one of them must vanquish the other. Reconciliation creates a gray zone of understanding that is necessary for psychological health. Unreconciled conflicts concerning which pole to chose are at the heart of your suicidal patient's world. The following are examples of these conflicts:

- Should I live or die?
- Am I being good or bad?
- Am I normal or abnormal?
- Am I in control or out of control?
- Should I approach or avoid emotional pain?
- Should I confront or hide from interpersonal conflict and rejection?
- Should I be passive or active?

Tunnel vision in suicidal crisis occurs when your patient is unable to see more than one pole at a time.

To use reconciling processes therapeutically, you need to understand that the tendency to search for the right meaning can be seductive both for your patient and for you. People in distress experience a temptation to decide on a particular kind of meaning to the exclusion of potentially opposite kinds of meanings. For example, a suicidal crisis is actually about living and dying, not the triumph of dying over living. To develop an affirmation of life, one must understand that life can and will produce desperately low moments. These two poles must simultaneously be in focus for effective behavioral and emotional functioning. This work is difficult for a therapist who is feeling pressure to do something constructive and optimistic in the midst of a suicidal crisis. Sometimes the most effective moments of therapy occur when you as the therapist are able to model an acceptance of these competing forces.

When your suicidal patient indicates that the current level of suffering is unacceptable, he or she is in effect rejecting both the reality and validity of simultaneously experiencing pain and pleasure. Any individual who consistently fails to accept these opposites runs grave risk of engendering tremendous amounts of suffering, because there is no balance that the individual can attain when suffering is present. Both you and your patient need to understand that the dilemma is in how to be both in control and out of control. By letting go of control, suicidal patients can attain balance. Control is the problem, not the solution.

The goal of establishing balance through reconciliation of seemingly polarized states is essential not only for the immediate suicidal crisis but also for developing a more robust adaptation to subsequent periods of pain and suffering. For example, when you teach your patient to look at all sides of the issue when describing an experience, you are teaching an acceptance of opposites. When you join experiences that look mutually contradictory and help your patient make room for each, your patient learns that both can coexist within the same human being; one does not have to vanquish the other. In the linear mode, this attitude is referred to as the ambivalence of the patient about dying; in the reconciling mode, these concepts are life and death resonating against each another. We leave it to you to figure out which explanation sounds like a problem and which sounds like a resolution.

The Role of Suicidal Behavior in Therapy

You are inviting failure if the sole goal of therapy is to prevent suicidal behavior in your patient. If suicidal behavior occurs again after therapy has started, and it sometimes does, you may feel both defeated by and angry at your patient. An alternative view is that there is continuity between real life and therapy that will not change because your patient has entered treatment. There is little reason to believe that most individuals will stop being suicidal simply because they come in to your presence. It is helpful to remember the old saying "It is much better to ride in the same direction as the horse." Avoid defining the context as one in which success is measured by whether the patient does or does not think about or attempt suicide. Make it crystal clear that the recurrence of suicidal behavior is regrettable, but do not assume that the very problem the patient is seeking help for will disappear solely as a consequence of entering treatment. If that were true, the act of entering treatment would be the treatment. We could discharge every patient after (or perhaps before) the first contact. Beware of the dilemma your rescue fantasies can produce. Members of our profession do not take kindly to people who are reluctant to be rescued. Working with a suicidal person rarely involves an instant save. Your first task is to get down to the hard work of developing a consistent, honest, and caring approach.

The Initial Contact: Evaluation Is Part of Treatment

Table 5–2 presents the most important goals and strategies of the initial meeting with a suicidal patient. These goals and strategies are valid whether the contact is the first in a series of repeated therapeutic contacts, a one-time session for generating a referral, or a crisis management session.

The Main Objectives

The objectives of the treatment session are to reframe suicidal behavior as problem-solving behavior and to provide the assurance and emotional support the patient needs. There is usually a sense of urgency and difficulty. The goal is to form a working relationship with your patient and to respond to the

Table 5–2.   Goals and strategies of the initial session with the suicidal patient

Goals	Strategies
1. Reduce the patient's fear about suicidality.	1A. "Normalize" suicidal behavior.
	1B. Legitimize feeling suicidal in the current context.
	1C. Talk about different forms of suicidal behavior calmly and openly.
2. Reduce the patient's sense of emotional isolation.	2A. Validate the patient's sense of pain.
	2B. Form collaborative set with patient.
	2C. Validate the presence of the three *I*s.
	2D. Look for competent social supports.
3. Activate problem solving in the patient.	3A. Reframe suicidal behavior as problem-solving behavior.
	3B. Isolate any spontaneous positive problem solving and praise it.
	3C. Develop idea of studying suicidal behavior in the context of problem solving.
	3D. Form short-term positive action plan (3–5 days).
4. Provide emotional and problem-solving support until follow-up care is engaged.	4A. Form crisis card with patient (see Chapter 7, "Managing Suicidal Emergencies").
	4B. Schedule support call.
	4C. Initiate medication regimen when appropriate.
	4D. Set follow-up appointment or give patient a referral.

many concerns that go along with a potentially explosive situation. At this initial meeting, you need to attend to simple realities. Documentation of various aspects of suicidality is important (see Appendix D, Suicidal Thinking and Behaviors Questionnaire). However, there is not much likelihood that either a brilliant maneuver or a bad gaffe will prevent or precipitate a suicide, respectively. The odds against your patient's dying by suicide are high, and risk factors are of little use to you in predicting your patient's behavior, especially in the short run. Accordingly, the definition of a quality contact is not simply keeping your patient alive but the degree to which you begin to collaborate on building better solutions in your patient's life.

The Checking-Out Process

The checking-out process can be the most dominant characteristic of the initial encounter with a suicidal patient. Your patient is ascertaining your attitudes about suicide. Do you label suicide as abnormal, do you become anxious or upset, or do you seem to accept it and move on? Your patient is checking to see what you do about suicidal behavior per se. Are you going to take an invasive, directive approach or a less invasive, more tolerant approach? Most important, your patient is checking to see whether you seem comfortable talking about and dealing with his or her sense of desperation.

The Desperate Clinician

Some clinicians experience a form of desperation in this initial session: a sense of needing to do something definitive or risk losing the patient. This feeling in itself creates a sense of anxiety within this initial session. Your patient can be extremely sensitive to signs of discomfort on your part. In the worst case, a nervous, pressured therapist creates a nervous, pressured client. Your composure and confidence are at least as important as the content of the interventions agreed to in the first meeting. Although there is an impact associated with using specific techniques, it is better to have a relaxed, matter-of-fact, calm clinician using a few techniques than a nervous, jittery, anxious clinician using many techniques.

Validation of Emotional Pain

A key outcome of the initial encounter is to validate your patient's emotional pain. Ascertain quite early in the interview how your patient feels and what problems are producing these feelings. At the first interview, the suicidal patient is often preoccupied with negative feelings and has a limited sense of problem-solving options. You must help your patient begin to understand and become more comfortable with emotional distress. The best way to give this assistance is to have your patient talk about the life circumstances involved in the crisis. Even if your patient is chronically suicidal, there are usually precipitating events, however trivial, that have recently increased emotional pain and desperation. As you listen, take the opportunity to produce empathetic statements about the patient's sense of desperation but without necessarily agreeing that the situation is indeed unsolvable. Here is an example of such a response: "The problems you have told me of are difficult ones. Almost anyone in your position would feel depressed and angry."

Validating emotional pain can be made more difficult if you are eager to rescue. Beware of your tendency to jump over the patient's pain and get to the business of finding solutions and saving people. This tendency is a frequent cause of negative outcome in the first encounter. Remember, the patient must understand that you believe feeling suicidal is a valid, understandable response to emotional pain. When a patient's pain is not being acknowledged, the patient may elevate the pain message to the point that it drowns out all subsequent activities in the session. In the worst case, the patient's suicidal potential may increase because the expressive component of the suicidal crisis has been downplayed or ignored. Tactics such as suggesting that the patient's level of emotional pain is not justified by the facts or that the patient has a lot to be thankful for (i.e., life is better than you think it is) are almost guaranteed to produce losing results.

The Problem-Solving Framework

Another major objective of the first encounter is to establish a problem-solving framework. Your use of language is critical. The way in which problems are reframed will help establish a clear connection between failed problem solving and suicidal behavior. Avoid making judgments about whether your patient has truly tried to solve problems. Accept that the patient's prior attempts to solve problems may have met with limited success. At the same time, acknowledge that your patient views suicidal behavior as a legitimate problem-solving option. Otherwise, suicidality would not be part of the crisis. Even if your patient is ambivalent about following through with suicidal behavior, that ambivalence is no different from the ambivalence associated with pursuing any other solution. All solutions have positive and negative consequences associated with them, and to a certain degree, all solutions produce some level of ambivalence. The following clinical encounter illustrates how to use information to reframe a patient's difficulties within a problem-solving context.

Therapist: What brings you in here today?

Patient: I've really been having a hard time lately. I've lost my job, and I'm not getting along well with my wife, and we've been talking about separating. I don't know where I'd live if we did separate, and I'm not sure that I could stand losing her.

Therapist: How does that make you feel?

Patient: Well, I go from feeling really anxious about what's going to happen to figuring that there's no hope and it's all going to end up bad. The reason I came here is because I've been thinking more and more about just ending it all. This is really starting to get scary. I've never felt this way before, and I'm beginning to wonder if I have control over what I'm going to do.

Therapist: It sounds like the situation is really difficult for you; there are lots of big losses and big question marks in your life. You're experiencing a lot of painful feelings, I can tell. I'm curious, would you say that suicide would be one way of solving these problems?

Patient: Well, I'm just tired of feeling bad; that's all I know.

Therapist: What is it about your attempt to solve these problems up to now that has led you to feel so bad?

Patient: Well, everything I've tried with my wife hasn't really changed the situation, and I don't see any prospect of getting work. I've put in several job applications, and all I keep getting is noes.

Therapist: So you're feeling really desperate because nothing you've tried with your partner seems to be working, and there's no prospect in sight for getting a new job. That must bring up a lot of fears about being alone and not having money.

Patient: Yeah, it sure does, and I'm not going to live my life that way.

Therapist: So, what you're saying is that if you can't solve these problems, you'd rather be dead than to live the life you imagine unfolding in front of you.

Patient: Yeah, that's pretty much it.

In the dialogue, the therapist both institutes a problem-solving set and validates the patient's sense of emotional desperation. In this brief example there is less emphasis on suicidal ideation as the problem and more emphasis on the patient's view of suicide in the problem-solving context. This strategy allows you to avoid a showdown over the validity of suicidal problem-solving options while at the same time joining with your patient's desperation around feeling bad and seeing no way out. Giving the patient permission to feel desperate and to see suicide as a potential option (even if it is not the best option) has an ameliorative impact on your patient's sense of crisis. In the example, the patient is scared by the occurrence of suicidal ideation in the first place. Creating a problem-solving frame of reference tends to defuse the self-control issue inherent in suicidal crisis. The problem-solving frame provides a different way of looking at the occurrence of suicidal behavior and allows your patient to take some distance from it, to step back and view the distressful event in a longer-term context. This movement of suicidality from an immediate distressful state to an understandable attempt to solve problems is a fundamental aspect of working with the suicidal patient during crisis.

Another way to establish a problem-solving set is to use humor. Although you should avoid humor that condescends to the patient or belittles emotional pain, it is often effective to use a play on words or a pun in relation to suicide. Your sense of humor in such circumstances has a way of defusing the seriousness attached to the crisis. For example, you might end a session by saying, "I was just reading a study yesterday that conclusively showed that all treatment is ineffective with dead clients. I thought you might like to know." Use humor in a manner that implies your confidence in your patient's ability to exercise self-control and get through the problem. This strategy can destabilize the patient's rigid cognitive framework and can be an important way of challenging any one of the three *I*s.

Talking Openly About Suicide

A most desired outcome in the first contact is to establish that it is okay to talk matter-of-factly, directly, and openly about suicide and that there is a credible framework that explains how suicidal behavior can occur. This framework will provide an alternative to the patient's operating concepts. Our patients usually walk in the door thinking that suicidality involves only mental illness, laziness, personal inadequacy, and loss of self-control.

Ending the Initial Session

The initial encounter should end with a plan of attack formulated and agreed to by you and your patient. This plan may involve an arrangement for your patient to contact another provider or to have a follow-up session. In this formulation, it is essential that you focus on small tasks rather than develop elaborate assignments. It is far more important for the patient to experience a small success than it is to strive for rarely obtained miracles. Often it is helpful to ask, If we could select a small task that, if you accomplished it, would tell you that things were just a little better, what would that be? Together the two of you may form an activities plan that will change your patient's unrewarding daily routine or accomplish a specific task that is viewed as a positive step forward. If you plan a follow-up appointment, consider the use of a self-monitoring activity to increase your patient's ability to observe natural fluctuations in emotional states. This task includes both negative states, such as hopelessness, intolerance of emotional pain, and suicidal ideation, and positive states, such as humor, appreciation of beauty in the surroundings, and kindly thoughts.

In Chapter 7 ("Managing Suicidal Emergencies") we discuss case management and crisis intervention techniques. Many of the strategies in that chapter are part of the concluding moments of this initial contact if your patient is continuing treatment with you. These strategies include steps such as setting up a crisis protocol with the patient, agreeing to an after-hours emergency protocol, and regular self-monitoring. Encourage your patient to focus on any moments between now and the next session when the situation seems to spontaneously be just a little bit better. Encourage your patient to be sensitive to spontaneous positive occurrences and at the same time to be aware of the fact that there will likely be a continuation of negative emotions. If your patient is going to see another provider, summarize together the key ingredients of the initial contact with special emphasis on what your patient thought was helpful. This information should be carefully relayed to the next provider so as to increase continuity of care.

The Early Phase of Treatment

The main goals and strategies for the continuation of treatment with a suicidal patient are listed in Table 5–3. The principal points to be addressed in the early phase of treatment are to install and reinforce a problem-solving set in your patient, to develop the patient's sense of competency to deal with emotional pain, and to begin solving problems in the real world. Remember, the essence of the suicidal patient's dilemma is being exposed to severe life obstacles that tax coping resources while at the same time making assumptions about the role of suffering that paralyzes an adaptive response.

Table 5–3. Goals and strategies in continuing treatment with the suicidal patient

Goals	Strategies
1. Destigmatize suicidal behavior.	1A. Develop personal scientist climate.
	1B. Use self-monitoring assignments.
	1C. Teach situational approach.
2. Objectify the patient's suicidal behavior.	2A. Use problem-solving reframing.
	2B. Provide ongoing validation of emotional pain– suicidal behavior relationship.
	2C. Move suicidal behavior off center.
	2D. Calmly and directly discuss past, present, and likely future of suicidal behavior.
3. Address likelihood of recurrent suicidal behavior.	3A. Develop agreements with patient about after-hours and other unplanned contacts and a behavioral crisis protocol.
	3B. Reaffirm that crisis card is workable.
	3C. Formulate a crisis management plan with likely contact points.
4. Activate problem-solving behavior in the patient.	4A. Teach personal problem-solving skills.
	4B. Develop better understanding of short-term versus long-term consequences.
	4C. Look for spontaneously occurring problem-solving behavior and praise it.
	4D. Set up small, positive problem-solving plans.
	4E. Teach specific skills necessary for better personal or interpersonal functioning.
5. Develop emotional pain tolerance in the patient.	5A. Approach suicide as an emotional avoidance behavior.
	5B. Teach distinction between just having and getting rid of feeling.
	5C. Instill contextual approach to negative thoughts and emotions.
	5D. Use acceptance exercises to teach distancing skills.
	5E. Emphasize experiential contact with emotional willingness versus suffering.
6. Develop specific interpersonal and problem-solving skills.	6A. Develop interpersonal skills.
	6B. Develop problem-solving skills.

Table 5–3.   Goals and strategies in continuing treatment with the suicidal patient *(continued)*

Goals	Strategies
7. Develop intermediate-term life direction.	7A. Use "What do you want your life to stand for?" exercise.
	7B. Discuss commitment to living life with negative thoughts and feelings.
	7C. Emphasize the process of striving for goals over the importance of reaching goals.
	7D. Set up intermediate-term goals and concrete, positive initial steps.
8. Terminate treatment with appropriate follow-up support.	8A. Develop relapse prevention plan.
	8B. Agree to a session-tapering schedule.
	8C. Reframe longer between-session intervals as "field trials."
	8D. Set up regular "booster" sessions.

Learning to Find Solutions

The immediate suicidal crisis may dissipate as a consequence of the first session, or it may continue into the next several sessions. In general, better-functioning patients—patients who are dealing with significant problems but have reasonable interpersonal skills—tend to resolve their crises faster than patients who have underlying character disorders. Regardless of the speed of resolution, the work in this phase of treatment is to develop an acceptance of the crisis per se and a commitment to find and act on solutions. Your specific strategy is twofold: to teach your patient how to make room for emotional pain and suffering as a way of minimizing the impact of pain and suffering and to get your patient to look at solutions other than suicide. Your treatment philosophy is always that there may well be better solutions; at the same time, you continue to be open to discussing suicide as an option your patient may continue to consider. Never create a situation in which your patient is uneasy discussing suicide with you.

Assaulting the Stigma

From the initial session to the end of treatment, you must continue to assault the stigma associated with suicidal behavior. Your patient will often continue to harbor secret thoughts that suicidal ideation or behavior is abnormal, cannot be accepted, and represents some form of personal weakness. Work constantly to show your patient that the weekly hassles that lead to increased suicidal ideation can be integrated into the problem-solving model. The idea is to help your patient see the flow of events that start from a bad situation, build into a sense of frustration or blockage, and end with the development of suicidal ideation. Therapy shifts attention from suicidal behavior per se to problem-solving behaviors that worked or did not work, or were not tried, before the emergence of suicidality. Your patient learns over time that suicidal behavior is a natural offshoot of ineffective problem solving, especially when intense emotional duress is present. Suicidal behavior is not something intrinsically bad. It is an attempt to solve a problem.

Situational Specificity

Your patient should learn the concept of situational specificity, a hallmark of cognitive-behavioral interventions. Specific situations tend to elicit particular and unique cognitive, emotional, and behavioral responses. Many of these responses are conditioned and may have outlived their usefulness. This concept is an assumption that suicidality is never experienced at a steady-state level. Instead, upswings in suicidal behavior are related to specific situations. These situations may appear trivial to the outside observer, but interpretive weight—the sense of meaning attached to them by your patient—makes the situations critical determinants of daily functioning. A clinically depressed patient may see a piece of burnt toast as a symbol of all that is wrong with his or her life; a suicidal patient can envision similarly trivial events in the same way. This feeling is not the province of depression; it is the province of individuals who are not adapting well, who are frustrated and in pain.

Self-Monitoring

Self-monitoring refers to the act of collecting information about one's thoughts, feelings, and behavior. These assignments are an elegant way of making a connection between the therapy process and the patient's real-life suicidal behavior without inadvertently overfocusing on suicidal behavior. You may ask your patient to keep a log of daily suicidal ideation with an intensity rating attached to it. This exercise allows the patient to see firsthand that suicidal ideation may fluctuate dramatically from hour to hour. Another instrument of considerable utility is a daily positive events diary compiled at the end of each day. The patient lists strategies that seemed to work reasonably well that day. This type of self-monitoring helps your patient refocus attention on things that work well as opposed to things that are problematic. These strategies are designed to destabilize your patient's notions about what is wrong and to help the patient develop a new outlook on suicidal behavior.

Through the therapeutic process, your patient learns to identify situations that tend to trigger emotional distress or lead to reduced tolerance of distress. Patterns usually begin to appear that reveal both underlying vulnerabilities and positive coping resources. Table 5–4 is a typical self-monitoring form that targets episodes of increased suicidal ideation.

Trigger Situations

The situation in Table 5–4 is an example of a trigger situation. It seems to involve the patient's spouse but is not generalized to similar situations with co-workers. The patient's answers may suggest that he has assumptions about the unacceptability of being criticized or abandoned by someone close. To use effective problem solving, the patient must learn to break these situations into bite-sized pieces. Trying to cope with feeling rotten all the time is an overwhelming task. Redressing a specific situation that produces emotional pain is more within the realm of possibility. You and your patient can role-play the situation and experiment with alternative strategies for managing negative feelings.

With self-monitoring assignments, set the situation so that it is difficult for your patient to fail. Beware of edicts such as "You should make entries in your log at least two or three times a day." Accept the patient's reports and use them in a positive way. When your patient sees that more systematic reporting would be useful, he or she will likely increase the number of entries. Some clinicians stumble badly around the issue of homework with suicidal patients and take compliance to be a measure of the patient's willingness to get better (i.e., resistance). Your general rule is to make sure that homework is seen as relevant by the patient and is packaged in bite-sized bits so that the patient cannot fail. For example, if the patient indicates reluctance to keep a written record, you might say, "You know, there are two types of people in the world: people who make lists and people who don't. Figure out which type you are, and collect the information in a way that works for you." If necessary, let the patient keep mental notes. Even if your patient brings in a seemingly trivial

Table 5–4. Sample weekly suicidal behaviors diary

Instructions: Each time you have a significant increase in suicidal ideation, please complete each of the columns below. Try to answer each column to help us understand your suicidal behavior.

Date	Situation	Negative thoughts	Negative feelings (rate standability 1–100)	Suicidal thoughts/ behavior (rate intensity and episode length (1–100)	Other problem-solving attempts (rate workability (1–100)
5/4	Received a letter from wife's attorney requesting property accounting.	1. She's going to clean me out—I won't be able to go through this.	Fear (20)	I don't want to go on with this. (60)	Took a long walk (45 minutes). (30)
		2. She lied to me about trying to work it out. I was a sucker to ever believe it.	Anger (30)	I just keep feeling worse and worse. (70)	Talked to my lawyer. (70)
		3. I will be alone again; maybe it's for the better.	Guilt (50)	At least my children would get insurance if I did it right. (30)	Tried to reach my brother but failed. (0)
			Loneliness (70)	There's no reason for waiting. (10) Length: 2 hours (80)	Tried to look at the bright side. (5)

mental note, heap praise on the patient and use the material.

An important and empowering goal in the early phase of treatment is to help your patient recognize which coping responses are working and which are not. It is easier to get a patient to enlarge on existing skills than it is to teach new problem-solving skills. Even the actively suicidal patient is solving some problems in daily life. Unfortunately, the patient's perceptual set and associated self-talk are focused on what is not working, and, accordingly, effective problem-solving efforts are overlooked. Your job is to help balance the picture by focusing on and reinforcing efforts that are succeeding. Using the problem-solving model, you can avoid making value judgments simply by asking the patient to rate whether a particular coping strategy has seemed to work.

For example, you can ask in a direct, somewhat curious way whether thinking about suicide in a specific situation worked as well as the patient might have hoped. The patient may reply immediately that thinking about suicide seemed to work better than just feeling bad, then on reflection the patient may indicate that suicidal thinking did not really work for more than a few minutes. Mention that there seem to be both short-term and long-term consequences that accompany any problem-solving behavior. This technique may help your patient to increase coping behaviors that are working reasonably well and at the same time begin an evaluation of behaviors that are frustrating and not solving anything. Praise spontaneous occurrences of effective problem solving and build on the patient's strengths. As your patient feels more competent, effective, and "response able" (see Chapter 6, "The Repetitiously Suicidal Patient," Allow Your Patient "To Be"), stressful situations become inherently less intolerable, interminable, and inescapable.

The Personal Scientist

The early phase of treatment is enhanced when you use the personal scientist approach, an approach basic to the cognitive-behavioral model of treatment (Beck et al. 1979). Ask your patient to try out the mind-set of being a scientist investigating his or her own behaviors. This approach can help your patient study problems, collect critical pieces of information for the evaluation process, and then modify responses according to the input. Your patient can collect data between sessions to test certain ideas. Emphasize developing responses that *do* work as opposed to responses that *ought to* work. When a new response is tried out, have your patient view it as an experiment. Experimentation means, you explain, that the response may not work. All problem-solving activities are viewed as endeavors that might need revision and change. There is no emphasis on success and failure. Remember, the recurrence of suicidal behavior is always labeled as an opportunity to investigate what worked and what did not work with a specific problem. At a deeper level, the balance inherent in this approach (focusing on both strengths and weaknesses) makes it an important component of the treatment process.

Three Clinical Pitfalls of the Early Phase of Treatment

The first common pitfall in the early part of treatment is to inadvertently focus the process of therapy on the presence versus absence of suicidal behavior. This initial suicidality often is quite intense, even though it may be of very brief duration. You may respond to this intensity by loading up on interventions designed to prevent suicidal behavior, the unintended result being narrowing the focus of therapy. In your efforts, you need to maintain an effective balance between intervening with the suicidal behavior and setting the stage for the broader range of interventions that will occur later.

The second pitfall is that you may try to move faster than your patient's condition will allow. You need to remember that a principal motivation of the patient may be to please others and be accepted. With all the urgency surrounding the suicidal crisis, your patient may mislead you about his or her actual level of functioning. To avoid this pitfall, you must constantly check out interventions with your patient. If there is any indication that your patient finds the tasks difficult, help trim the interventions down to bite-sized bits. This process gives your patient permission to go slow and makes it clear that you are quite happy with a pace that allows for a thorough understanding of what is transpiring. You are not interested in the speed of change. Your main concern is your patient's capacity to understand how change occurs and to build on that capacity.

The third pitfall is the halo effect, a phenomenon whereby your patient automatically reports doing better partly because of the halo or positive context of seeking therapy. This effect can produce a brief period of improvement, but the improvement can be followed by a strong rebound into suicidal crisis. The halo effect can catch you by surprise and lead to conflict, confrontation, and premature termination of treatment. The key intervention is to be positive about positive change but at the same time acknowledge that learning is an irregular process. A train never leaves the station smoothly. It always starts with bumps and jerks. This analogy is handy for this process (maybe your patient can think of a better one). Accept that functioning may be worse this week than it was the last week and do so in a way that does not make it appear that you are abandoning optimism about progress over time. Remind your patient that even though things are going better right now, he or she should not be surprised if some of the same problems resurface in the near future. Emphasize the importance of working with both positive and less-positive outcomes in the overall learning process.

Session Logistics and Course of Treatment

It is common practice to see a suicidal patient more often early in therapy and then to have regular, less-frequent sessions as the situation stabilizes. This approach may inadvertently encourage your patient to stay in crisis because more of your attention is forthcoming in that circumstance. The decision about session frequency must be geared to your patient's longer-term functioning and the degree to which the suicidal crisis is likely to respond to more intensive treatment. You may have to address the patient's fear about going an entire week without any contact with you. In addressing (problem solving) these fears, you may schedule an additional session or set up a telephone contact at a specific time midway through the week. In general, the more chronic the suicidal behavior, the less one should use additional session scheduling. An important goal with patients with chronic suicidal behavior is to teach emotional tolerance. This goal will be reached when your patient realizes that regular sessions are helpful and that the distress experienced between sessions can be tolerated and somewhat mastered. With better-functioning patients, use one or two sessions a week in the acute phase if clinical benefits accrue. The usual session frequency is once weekly. The number of sessions can be decreased to one every other week as the situation stabilizes and your patient is able to conduct more and more fieldwork and personal scientist activities between sessions. There is actually a benefit in scheduling biweekly sessions. It takes time to collect data about situational triggers; many of the important situations do not occur weekly.

There is no preset length of time or number of sessions associated with the initial phase of treatment. Some patients will move through this phase in one or two sessions, whereas other patients may take months. Three factors signal the end of the initial treatment phase. First, your patient develops acceptance and spontaneous use of the problem-solving mind-set in session. Second, your patient is secure in the knowledge that you understand his or her sense of desperation and pain. Third, your patient shows evidence of experimentation with problem-solving strategies in the field. These attempts may seem rudimentary, but good-faith efforts to use alternative strategies for dealing with stress and emotional pain in the real world mean your patient has moved to the next phase of treatment.

The Intermediate Phase of Treatment: Developing Acceptance of Feelings and a Commitment to Act

Every crisis provides an opportunity, and the depth of a suicidal crisis is an opportunity for your patient to develop a better understanding of suffering and its role in the experience of the world. Many people who have worked through suicidal behavior describe what they have learned in these terms. They see themselves as individuals with a greater capacity to tolerate a variety of emotional states. The primary goal during the intermediate phase of treatment is to help your patient develop a tolerance for emotionally distressing events. The focus is on learning that emotional pain can be tolerated and brought to a resolution. Your patient needs to understand that the meaning of events, and, importantly, suffering associated with these events, is produced in the private realm of his or her own thoughts, feelings, and thoughts about feelings. Emotional distress is a direct result of accepting only one way of thinking about things. Think of this situation as your patient's attaching to certain "hot" cognitions. Low tolerance arises when these hot cognitions refer to the unacceptability of feeling bad. For example, many hopelessness cognitions are hot because they raise provocative implications about suffering (i.e., there is no purpose in staying alive if one has to suffer). In this mode your patient can experience depression, anxiety, despair, sadness, and, eventually, suicidal ideation in relation to these thoughts.

Two major therapeutic models can be followed during the intermediate phase of therapy. The more conventional route is to use *cognitive therapy* to help your patient develop more realistic self-talk about either the life events or the negative feelings that occur in relation to life events. This approach is more traditional and culture supported because it relies on logic as a way to change your patient's thinking, feeling, and behaving. The suicidal patient is always a victim of taking a particular stand with regard to a difficult life situation. The phenomenon of tunnel vision is not limited to the suicidal depressive patient but is a characteristic of suicidal patients in general. You and your patient should work collaboratively to uncover critical cognitive errors and to construct field tests of their validity. In cases in which your patient clearly agrees there is a distorted interpretation, he or she can experiment with a more reasonable interpretation and see whether it works better the next time the situation occurs. Many of the deeper assumptions that indirectly or directly lead to suicide as a viable option can be examined by the patient and the clinician. To learn more about this approach, study the work of Beck et al. (1979).

A second approach, and one we often favor, is to develop an *acceptance of emotional pain* through the use of distancing and of nonevaluative self-observation strategies. The goal in this approach is to learn to make room for distressing thoughts and feelings while doing what needs to be done to respond to the demands of the outside world. There are two key strategies for increasing acceptance of uncomfortable emotions and thoughts. First, *recontextualization* is the process of teaching your patient to look at the relationship of thoughts, feelings, and behaviors in a way that provides more options for handling problems. Second, the act of *comprehensive distancing* involves stepping back from one's thoughts and feelings and looking at them as an observer rather than a participant.

Recontextualization

Each day brings all of us an incredible array of thoughts and feelings. Humans process literally thousands of cognitive and emotional experiences daily, usually with only minimal awareness. These processes are not unconscious because they can be accessed directly through voluntary shifts of attention. The processes are better thought of as automatic conditioned responses. Many of us tend to treat thoughts and feelings as if they were literal substitutes for experience; that is, cognitions and emotions are put in a position of being at least as real as the situations that are responsible for them.

For people in both acute and chronic crises, thoughts and feelings take on a consistently negative overtone. The relationship your patient establishes with negative thoughts can be viewed as the cause of suffering. The analogy to use is the distinction between chronic pain and disability. Some people are able to live with chronic pain by realizing they have new limitations and the job is to carry on with life. They accept the pain and continue their life's work, embracing challenges as they come. Other persons with chronic pain, however, see pain as a reason why life cannot go on, at least not until a cure is produced that will get rid of the pain. Many people in the grip of these chronic pain emotions and cognitions seem fixed on the idea that such a cure is somehow, somewhere available, and they suspend many aspects of their lives as they search, often futilely, or wait, often angrily, for relief. For these persons, pain becomes a reason for not working, not participating in family life, and avoiding intimacy. Their pain experiences usually worsen, and the person becomes disabled. This person does not accept pain, and the pain becomes the dominant theme in the person's life—a life that becomes increasingly less satisfying.

To be suicidal, a person must be unwilling to accept emotional pain and must see suicidal behavior as a way to get rid of unacceptable thoughts and feelings. Pain avoidance may be why suicidal behavior and other consciousness-numbing avoidance behaviors, such as alcohol use, drug use, and eating disorders, tend to occur together. All these behaviors serve the same purpose: to take the edge off pain. When acceptance is low, most of the person's resources are spent trying to eliminate suffering rather than making adaptive changes in behavior. Like the functionally disabled pain patient, the suicidal patient is not doing what needs to be done to adapt to life's circumstances and uses language that implies negative thoughts and feelings are responsible (causes) for the dysfunction.

The objective of recontextualization is not to get rid of disturbing thoughts or feelings but to teach the patient to make room for them and do what needs to be done to get on with life. The objective is met when your patient learns that negative thoughts or feelings do not block adaptive behavior. The two can coexist. Needed behavior change can occur even in the presence of ongoing suicidal ideation and emotional distress. Your patient can learn how to accept negative private events without excessive self-evaluation. When the thought-feeling-behavior relationship has been recontextualized, your patient does not need to engage in a contest to see whether suicidal thinking can be eliminated or whether the urge to follow through on the thought can be resisted. When you encourage your patient to bring negative, ambivalent, and positive feelings into the problem-solving process while at the same time remaining committed to change, the patient learns that tolerance for emotional distress means seeing distressful thoughts and feelings for what they are (a covert influence on the way one behaves), not what they advertise themselves to be (monsters waiting to devour us if we allow them in the house).

Comprehensive Distancing

The act of comprehensive distancing is accomplished when your patient establishes a willingness to detach from active participation in suicidal thoughts or affective distress. A powerful strategy is the *dual-thermometer exercise.* Have your patient keep a daily diary, rating two dimensions of experience on a 1–10 scale at the end of each day. The first scale is a *willingness thermometer,* describing a noncritical openness to have whatever experiences occur during the day. This state is best described as being present for, mildly interested in, and observant of these experiences. The other scale is a *suffering thermometer,* describing how much distress your patient feels in the presence of these experiences. Have the patient rate both scales each day, making short notes on any factors that seem associated with an increase or decrease on either scale compared with the previous day. The two thermometers will typically reveal an inverse relationship between willingness and suffering. In general, as willingness goes up, an active sense of suffering goes down. Use your patient's own positive experience with moments-of-willingness ratings as a jumping-off point to build *willingness skills.* These techniques help your patient develop a healthy skepticism about the usefulness of attaching to hot thoughts and feelings. For some better-functioning suicidal patients, increases on the willingness scale can occur in treatment, often with strong clinical results in one or two sessions.

An additional advantage of comprehensive distancing strategies is that you are able to use them to both monitor and use recurring suicidal ideation as part of treatment. A difficult clinical task at any stage of treatment is finding a way to be attentive to your patient's ongoing suicidal experiences without inadvertently making that the sole focus of clinical intervention. Once comprehensive distancing becomes a viable strategy, suicidal thinking or behavior can be framed as just another example of low acceptance of certain emotions. In other words, suicidal thinking is designed to get rid of, rather than make room for, negative feelings. Remember, even when other problems are the current focus of treatment, suicidal behavior can easily be brought back into the mainstream in the event of a crisis. Along with many highly useful therapeutic strategies, Hayes et al. (1999) provide a detailed formulation of acceptance as behavior change.

Personal Problem-Solving Skills

During the intermediate phase, you will want to help your patient develop specific skills that can increase adaptive social and interpersonal behavior. Specific behavioral skills training can be delivered during individual therapy sessions or in skills-training groups. We find that a particularly effective model is to combine skills-training groups with individual therapy sessions. This approach allows your patient to continue working on developing pain tolerance and problem-solving abilities individually while learning new skills in a supportive group environment. If skills training is delivered without work on acceptance, your patient may see the skills as a new, more sophisticated tactic for avoiding or eliminating emotional pain. In other words, the skills will be put in the service of the same self-defeating agenda as before. It is often helpful to say, "The reason we are focusing on these skills is that you have a job to do in life while you are in pain. The better you know these skills, the more likely it is you will use them even while you are hurting."

Effective personal problem solving evolves through several discrete stages: 1) problem identification, 2) identification of alternative problem-solving strategies, 3) evaluation of the likely utility of different problem-solving responses, 4) selection of a specific problem-solving technique and formation of a plan, and 5) implementation of the response and evaluation of the effects of the response. Deficits in any of these skill areas may put your patient at risk of lingering problems and chronic life stress. This pragmatic approach to personal problem solving underscores the empirical, trial-and-error nature of effective efforts at addressing life problems. Teach your patient the absolute necessity of using feedback in approaching life's difficulties. Feedback emphasizes a "no failure" aspect in that all problem-solving approaches are viewed as "best guesses." The process of problem solving must be done repetitively until enough information is obtained to effectively overcome the obstacle. Given the well-established problem-solving passivity of the suicidal individual, this model offers a concrete, teachable alternative that will give your patient the tools for performing in an active mode.

Even when the specifics of this model are being taught in a group or psychoeducational format, you can and must simultaneously work with your patient on beliefs that undermine proactive problem solving. The use of active problem-solving homework assignments will stimulate the patient's feelings of hopelessness, predictions of personal failure and abandonment, and many other performance-stopping beliefs. You can help the patient test some of these negative predictions through the use of highly structured homework assignments that are based on the problem-solving model.

Interpersonal Effectiveness

In the interpersonal skills arena, you should emphasize an approach that integrates interpersonal, social, and assertiveness skills. The three key components of interpersonal effectiveness are *conflict resolution skills, general social skills,* and *appropriate assertiveness.*

Conflict resolution skills generally emphasize finding a common ground on which a conflict with someone else can be worked out in a way that satisfies everyone's interests. Because of the suicidal patient's passive style and tendency to make black-and-white judgments, it is difficult for this person to imagine a resolution of some interpersonal conflict that would obtain the desired outcome, maintain the relationship, and enhance the patient's self-esteem. By learning negotiation skills, including techniques for developing a common best interest, your patient is more likely to steer this delicate course to an effective resolution. Again, a combination of individual therapy and skills-training groups is a very effective package. The therapist generally takes responsibility for working on personal issues associated with application of skills, and the group leaders focus on teaching basic component skills.

General social skills and *appropriate assertiveness* are important. These areas of functioning can be very difficult ones for the suicidal patient, who often has poor skills (e.g., does not maintain eye contact, apologizes instead of saying no) and very negative beliefs (e.g., "If I stand up for myself, my spouse will dump me"). When working with assertiveness skills, focus on the ability to maintain an assertive response in the face of strong opposition. The suicidal patient often lives in interpersonal environments marked by increased dysfunction and interpersonal conflict. The other players in this environment may not be particularly well put together either and may respond to healthy behavior with undermining, cajoling, or demeaning responses. It is important to confront the patient with these responses in skills-training groups so that the patient can develop a "thicker skin." There is often a person in your patient's social network who is routinely negative and problematic. Try to teach skills that will enable the patient to consistently set limits despite negative feedback from that dysfunctional person. The more realistically your patient is able to practice by role-playing, the better he or she will be able to handle the real event. It is useful to do role reversals in which the patient plays the role of the dysfunctional person and has to model the reactions the other person would have. The trainer takes on the role of the patient and models limit-setting responses.

There are excellent books that can be used as a guide to such training. We encourage you to consult these more comprehensive texts, some of which are listed in Selected Readings. It is important to realize that skill deficits are important determinants of your patient's suicidal behavior. Skill deficits may have occurred because of faulty training from a dysfunctional family, specific cultural deprivation or aberration, or just plain lack of available role models. The keys to forming better adaptive relationships are the presence of effective cognitive and emotional perspectives and the ability to act appropriately in one's environment (i.e., do what needs to be done when you need to do it).

Three Clinical Pitfalls of the Intermediate Phase of Treatment

The first major pitfall in the intermediate phase can be the tendency to *lose focus* once the acute suicidal crisis has passed. The principal symptom of this pitfall is a lack of session-to-session continuity and more of a "what's on your mind this week" approach. Clinicians often feel emotionally winded at this stage and prefer to let the patient direct the form and content of the therapy. This style is unfortunate, because this phase provides the opportunity to address key cognitive, emotional, and spiritual issues. The therapist's goal is to increase both the patient's problem-solving flexibility and the patient's problem-solving view of the world. The optimal time for reaching this goal is when your patient is not operating in the crisis mode.

A second pitfall is to assume that the absence of crisis means that suicidal behavior has stopped. This phase often involves the persistence of *chronic low-level suicidal ideation*. Because it does not represent a crisis, the ideation is not focused on in treatment. Chronic low-level suicidal ideation is an ideal target for work in the intermediate phase. Because the pain associated with such experiences is not so intense, it is easier to get your patient to experiment with tasks such as emotional pain tolerance, observational interventions, and personal problem-solving plans.

A third and more subtle pitfall is *negative countertransference,* which can be ironically linked to the patient's improvement. In other words, your need to rescue has been fulfilled and yet your patient has not finished therapy. This pitfall is dangerous if you begin to lose interest and become distracted. You can also begin to engage in subtle behaviors indicating a lack of commitment to continuing to the end of the treatment. It can look as if you are no longer concerned about your patient's quest to address different life problems. Because your attention is a powerful reinforcement, your patient may respond to this shift by resuming or escalating suicidal behavior.

Session Scheduling and Course of Treatment

The intermediate phase of therapy is more difficult to gauge in terms of both its beginning and its ending points. In general, this phase begins when the acute crisis has been defused to the point that the patient can talk about suicidal ideation, negative thoughts, and emotional distress as part of a single continuum. Some patients find it easier to adapt to this mindfulness approach, especially if they have had spiritual experiences such as prayer, meditation, or yoga that have given them some ability to be distant from and contemplate events. Patients with strong obsessional traits or highly rationalized defense styles tend to move more slowly into the acceptance and commitment model. These patients rigidly defend against their negative thoughts. Asking them to become more accepting can be perceived as quite dangerous (i.e., "If I let the thoughts in the house, they will burn it down."). Try to focus on developing split perspectives with such patients. With this strategy each thought sequence about an event is seen as a story. The exercise is to have your patient tell the story over and over, each time with a different connotation. Some endings can be better, some worse. The goal is not to keep going until the patient gets the right story but to have your patient experience the reality of there being multiple outcomes to an approach to any life or mental obstacle. This approach will often help the more obsessive patient accept the mindfulness approach.

The frequency of sessions during the intermediate phase can be quite variable. Sessions can be as much as 2 or 3 weeks apart to accommodate experiential learning. The sequencing between sessions also may be highly variable. For example, there may be times when weekly sessions are indicated followed by a phase in which meetings every 2 or 3 weeks are better suited to the patient's pace of change. In some settings, weekly sessions are not consistently available. A good plan is to move to a regular but less-frequent session schedule as soon as the acute crisis has been addressed. Try to collaborate with your patient on developing a schedule of sessions that makes sense, focusing on the work required between sessions and the amount of support your patient needs.

End of the Intermediate Phase

The intermediate phase of treatment ends when the patient truly understands and uses the treatment—the patient "gets it." Your patient is now reporting an *integrated perspective* that comes in the midst of situations that previously produced suicidal ideation. Look for situations in which your patient selects new problem-solving strategies even while acknowledging that the possibility of suicidal behavior occurred as one possible course of action. Another indicator is your patient's reporting that, even though many of the same thoughts and feelings are occurring, these thoughts and feelings do not seem as credible or as demanding as they once were. There are great variations among patients in movement through the intermediate phase of treatment. Higher-functioning patients may complete the work in 1 or 2 months. Chronically suicidal patients with character difficulties may need a year or more to integrate the concepts necessary to complete this part of treatment.

The Termination Phase of Treatment: Building the Future

The final phase in working with the suicidal patient is to develop a plan that addresses the longer-term needs of your patient and that has a built-in, self-correcting component for preventing relapse. At termination of treatment, your patient has established good problem-solving alternatives to suicidal behavior but knows that suicidal thinking may not have entirely disappeared. It is vital that your patient know that reemergence of suicidal ideation is a signal that low acceptance is present and old forms of avoidant problem solving are being used. Reoccurring suicidal thinking needs to be used as a stimulus for initiating acceptance strategies and committing to proactive problem-solving strategies.

Dealing With Dependency

Although termination is always an issue in successful treatment, it is perhaps more so with suicidal patients. Your patient has been through a crisis with you, and that simple fact creates a potential for dependency. Your patient may see you as a necessity, a major component of any future change. *Dependency must be dealt with in the termination phase.* It is important to lavish praise on your patient for effective problem-solving behaviors or spontaneous examples of heightened acceptance. Use explanations that discount the importance of therapy in this process and emphasize the many hours per week the patient is out of therapy. Point out that there is only 1 hour per week of treatment but 167 hours per week "in the field." It is vital that your patient develop the ability to feel good about handling tough situations. Your goal is to internalize the patient's self-praise and not to take credit for any changes that have occurred. At the same time, your patient has to accept that suicidal ideation could reappear and have a prevention plan for when that happens.

Shaping a Positive Future

Help your patient to identify the central features of a positive future and to begin shaping that future through goal setting. It is not an acceptable clinical outcome to simply weather a crisis and start out symptom free from the same basic spot in life. It is important to stimulate the patient to set valued life goals. One way to approach this is to ask, What do you want your life to stand for? If you were to die tomorrow, what would be the most important thing you would want to be remembered for? Get the patient to specify in concrete terms some intermediate goals that would represent steps in the right direction. In general, the suicidal patient is overfocused on outcome and tends to underplay the importance of process. Emphasize that attaining life goals may not be nearly as important as what is learned on the way toward reaching those goals. Patients often recall instances in which a goal is in sight, only to find it has been outgrown. In other words, the work of striving toward one's goals in the here and now is what life is all about. Applying this strategy with the chronically suicidal patient can be at the high end of the difficulty continuum, because these individuals may be all but completely absorbed in what has not been accomplished in life and may have great difficulty placing value on the hard work of goal setting and problem solving. Many patients have endured significant interpersonal or material losses as a consequence of their suicidal behavior. The idea of building for the future is very reassuring and allows for a constructive approach to what comes next.

The Role of Relapse Prevention

Preventing or reducing relapse potential is accomplished by preparing your patient for likely tests of his or her commitment to nonsuicidal problem solving. This step involves development of *early risk warning systems* and development of a clear *response plan* that incorporates skills and techniques that have already worked. It is helpful to dovetail this activity into the intermediate-term life-planning process. In this way, the potential recurrence of suicidal behavior can be reframed as one of many potential obstacles your patient will need to move through. It is important to tell your patient to expect a crisis and that this crisis will be an invitation to consider suicidal problem solving. Ask your patient to think carefully about the earliest signs of increasing suicidal potential. These signs may be social withdrawal, self-preoccupation (i.e., attaching more than the usual amount of energy to certain types of thoughts), and low acceptance of feelings. Walk through the process of treatment to identify which skills and techniques are most compatible with your patient's coping style. Encourage the use of skills and techniques that most closely match this style. Skills that are compatible with a patient's personality or world outlook are much more likely to be remembered and used than skills that seem artificial, contrived, or persistently uncomfortable to use. Rehearse the response plan and ask your patient to imagine any obstacles that might get in the way of implementing this plan. Have your patient imagine and rehearse strategies for overcoming the obstacles and then get to the point of implementing the response plan. Table 5–5 lists elements of a typical prevention and intermediate-term life plan.

Putting a New Frame on Terminating Treatment

Your patient should view termination of treatment as a process of field experiments built around a model of session tapering. This process involves decreasing session frequency in a sequence of progressively longer gaps. For

Table 5–5. Sample suicide prevention plan

1. What are the first signs of trouble in the way I believe, think, feel, or behave (e.g., sleeping less well, avoiding social situations, getting more depressed or anxious)?
   a.
   b.
   c.
   d.
2. How do I plan to monitor myself to watch for these signs? If I plan to watch for the above signs, when and how do I plan to check for them?
   If I plan to rate my suicidal thinking, when and how will I do this?
3. What are my most important goals for the next year?
4. What stresses do I anticipate in the next year, both ongoing (e.g., job problems, sick older parent) and new (e.g., move to a new house, Christmas at my house), and how do I plan to cope with them?
5. What is/are the most valuable idea(s) I have learned in treatment up to now, and how do I plan to remember it/them?
6. What is/are the most valuable coping strategies I have learned in treatment, and what and how and when do I plan to use it/them?
7. What hurdles might occur that would get in the way of using these coping strategies, and how would I overcome them (e.g., too tired to cope, get down on myself for having problems)?

example, a typical session-tapering schedule might involve meetings at 1, 2, 3, and 6 months. The goal in each meeting is to review the results of the previous field experiment with reference to the relapse prevention plan and life goals. Establishing prearranged meeting times allows the patient to return for a booster session even if his or her life is going very well. State that unscheduled visits are available, but encourage your patient to go as long and as hard as possible before making an unplanned visit. The fact that a scheduled session is already on the books is reassuring to the patient and tends to promote a sense of a safe environment in which to experiment with new pain tolerance and problem-solving strategies.

Ideally, your patient should terminate therapy. In the natural flow of the session-tapering model, your patient may suggest that a return visit really is not needed. This form of termination is optimal because your patient, rather than you, is initiating breaking the bond. On the other hand, some patients may want to stay connected, even at the level of checking in once a year. This system is an efficient use of your time and can be an important part of relapse prevention. In this scenario, your patient may not return for the yearly visit but may eventually contact you and want to discuss how things are going. In this case, immediately praise the patient for testing an even longer period than that originally scheduled.

Used properly, the session-tapering model decreases termination anxiety, enhances your patient's sense of autonomy, and keeps the door open for a return to therapy in a cost-effective way. Avoid the scenario of the suicidal patient's viewing terminating treatment as a test of whether the problem has been cured. This scenario can cause your patient to see a return to therapy because of suicidal thinking as an indication of failure. By developing a model that makes a suicidal crisis part of an ongoing learning paradigm, you can avoid situations in which the patient needlessly avoids treatment. Always be available for "tune-up" visits, and always emphasize that you can be much more helpful early in the game. It is more efficient to intervene early than to deal with a patient who returned to the suicidal mode some time ago and is struggling with an even greater sense of failure.

When your patient returns because of a setback, place the decision to come back into therapy in a positive context. Suggest that your patient has picked exactly the right time to come in for help. Express admiration for the courage and wisdom needed to make the decision. It is important to discuss the new crisis in a way that suggests it is a new learning situation and not the patient's failure to remember things past. Learning acceptance and problem-solving strategies is an incremental task. There are periods in which any of us will exhibit fewer skills than were evident the week before. Life challenges are complex and ever changing. It is not always clear to your patient how particular skills may apply, given the new properties of stressful situations. If your patient is willing to approach therapy early in the new suicidal crisis, it is often amazing how quickly crises are solved the second, third, or fourth time around. What has taken several weeks or months to achieve in the first episode of care is achieved in only one or two sessions. Go to great lengths to point out how quickly your patient seems to be responding to the need to apply new skills. In other words, always build self-efficacy when dealing with a relapse by your patient.

If your patient has simply not used the relapse prevention plan, you should avoid resistance interpretations. Instead, focus on obstacles that may have gotten in the way of implementing the plan. You should take the blame for failing to get a clear enough vision of the potential obstacles. Apologize and then work with the patient to troubleshoot the plan. The goal is to empower your patient to build a better future over time. This goal is met not through blaming but through shaping, practice, and reshaping.

Clinical Pitfalls of the Termination Phase of Treatment

The most important pitfall to avoid at the termination phase of treatment is creating a situation in which your patient feels abandoned and cut off by you. This situation is most likely to occur if you have not begun dealing with the issue of ending treatment early enough. Unfortunately, it is not unusual for a clinician to decide at the end of one session to end therapy at the conclusion of the next session. When this decision is made, the issue has not been integrated into the treatment process. A good general strategy is to discuss the time-limited nature of the therapy contract in the early part of the intermediate phase of treatment and to form agreements about how your patient and you will know that therapy can be moved into a field-experiment phase. The more directly or matter-of-factly this reality can be approached, the easier it will be to actually move to the field-trial and session-tapering phase.

A second pitfall is the development of a tacit understanding between the patient and therapist that the therapist's brilliance is responsible for the patient's clinical improvement. The patient begins to fear life without the therapist as the termination/field-trial phase nears. To avoid this pitfall, you should consistently put responsibility for positive changes back in the patient's lap. You can accomplish this task very effectively by being both pleased with and curious about the methods your patient uses to accomplish a variety of goals, even small ones, in the process of therapy. The emphasis in these discussions is to get your patient to accept the credit for what has happened and to make this progress a part of the patient's self-concept.

The heart of every therapist's rescue fantasy is the encounter with the eternally grateful patient who attributes miraculous properties to the therapist. To let go of ownership of miracles, you need to remain mindful of the real limits of personal persuasion and influence over others. The therapeutic community is somewhat to blame for this problem in promoting the idea that therapists cause patients to change. In Chapter 6 ("The Repetitiously Suicidal Patient"), we describe how this destructive mythology can play a prominent role in negative treatment outcomes. For the present, remember to take responsibility for all failures and give your patient credit for all successes. This stance is humbling; it is an ego-reducing exercise that will have long-term benefits for you. Most important, it works.

Conclusion

Conducting therapy with a suicidal patient is a complex process that often brings out the best and the worst in us. We have chosen disciplines that involve helping others, but what is helpful in this particular circumstance? The answer to that question is at the heart of many of the mixed feelings we have when working with acutely suicidal patients. It also explains the tremendous range of negative feelings elicited by the person who is unresponsive to and critical of our efforts, such as a chronically suicidal patient. Avoiding the temptation to promote treatment as a way of getting rid of emotional pain or disturbing thoughts seems like a good place to start. Unfortunately, our patients ask us to do just that. This task not only is impossible but also is an unrealistic portrayal of our contract with life. What we can do is help our patients focus on the inevitability of tragedies, setbacks, and personal failures as well as the joys and challenges of continuing into the future. We can help by being clear about the values that guide our understanding of life-and-death matters. Our most valuable resource is our capacity to respond to our patients' emotional pain. What will help lead our patients through the pain and into the future is our ability to collaborate and learn together. We should not assume that what we would do is automatically what our patients need to do. These decisions are a matter of individual discovery and can only be aided by our acceptance and commitment.

Helpful Hints

- The major goal of treatment of a suicidal patient is to change one or more of the three *I*s (pain that is intolerable, inescapable, and interminable).
- The problem-solving approach reframes suicidal behavior as a form of problem solving.

- Remember to always validate the patient's emotional pain.
- Focus on teaching the patient methods for tolerating emotional pain.
- Focus on using real-life problems to teach the patient better problem-solving skills.
- Use ongoing suicidal behavior as a jumping-off point to teach problem solving.
- Try to adopt a collaborative, personal scientist approach with the patient.
- Teach the patient that negative thoughts and feelings can be accepted and adaptive responses can still be made.
- Focus on developing interpersonal, problem-solving, self-control, and stress management skills in individual and group settings.
- Focus on reconciling conflicting beliefs that support the patient's ambivalence about life and living.

References

Beck A, Rush J, Shaw D, et al: Cognitive Therapy for Depression: A Treatment Manual. New York, Guilford, 1979

Hayes S, Strosahl K, Wilson K: Acceptance and Commitment Therapy: An Experiential Approach to Behavior Change. New York, Guilford, 1999

Selected Readings

Ascher M (ed): Paradoxical Procedures in Psychotherapy. New York, Guilford, 1989

de Shazer S: Clues: Investigating Solutions in Brief Therapy: An Experiential Approach to Behavior Change. New York, WW Norton, 1988

Jacobson N (ed): Psychotherapists in Clinical Practice: Cognitive and Behavioral Perspectives. New York, Guilford, 1987

Pollock LR, Williams JMG: Effective problem solving in suicide attempters depends on specific autobiographical recall. Suicide Life Threat Behav 31:386–396, 2001

Raes F, Hermans D, de Decker A, et al: Autobiographical memory specificity and affect-regulation: an experimental approach. Emotion 3:201–206, 2003

6

The Repetitiously Suicidal Patient

Evaluation, Psychotherapy, and
Basic Case Management

Few patients represent more of a challenge to mental health and medical practitioners than the repetitiously suicidal individual. Whether the suicidal behavior is repeated sublethal overdosing or near-lethal attempts at killing oneself seems to make little difference. Health care systems have difficulty in dealing with these patients, because the patients are a source of conflicts between providers. Practitioners often diagnose character disorders or personality disorders in these patients, and both terms are synonymous with trouble. These individuals can challenge a practitioner's theoretical and practical assumptions, and they can reveal gaps in service delivery systems. Repetitiously suicidal patients present their suicidality in a host of encounters within both the general health and mental health care systems. Emergency department physicians deal with and feel frustrated by these people as much as seasoned psychotherapists do. A primary care physician is as likely as an inpatient psychiatrist to feel overwhelmed by such a patient. In other words, there is something universal about the dilemma presented by this type of suicidal patient. The system response to a chronically suicidal patient often does not work well, partly because of a singular focus on suicide prevention and liability reduction that can limit effective treatment.

Although repetitiously suicidal patients often receive a clinical diagnosis of borderline personality disorder, it is probably more appropriate to describe them as multiproblem patients because of the widespread deficiencies in their cognitive, emotional, behavioral, and social functioning. Such patients typically experience long-term difficulties with a variety of negative emotional states, such as depression, anxiety, apathy, boredom, loneliness, guilt, and anger. This chronic negative affect is a major driver of a plethora of maladaptive coping responses, chief among them being repetitious suicidal behavior, and addictive behaviors, such as alcohol and drug abuse, eating disorders, and chronic self-mutilation. Multiproblem patients also experience significant difficulties in social and interpersonal functioning. They have trouble forming and maintaining interpersonal relationships and frequently inject the therapy process with a conflict-laden set of issues around forming and maintaining both casual and intimate adult relationships. Multiproblem patients often report inconsistent work histories and typically do not utilize social supports in the community, such as friends, family, church, and community resources.

At the level of daily living, multiproblem patients maintain a precarious balance between tolerating chronic, aversive mental events (i.e., depression, self-critical thinking, traumatic memories, and anxious rumination) and meeting the minimal requirements for routine social functioning. When internal or external events trigger heightened levels of negative affect, multiproblem patients may exhibit dissociative behavior or frank psychotic symptoms, such as hallucinations and delusional thinking. The multiproblem patient often engages in a sedentary and isolated lifestyle that results in excessive time spent in self-focused attention. At the same time, the patient has difficulty tolerating and regulating the aversive mental states that are the outgrowth of self-focused awareness. This self-regulatory failure, and the extreme coping responses it provokes, is a core feature of the high-risk behavior patterns that providers often struggle with when working with such patients.

Therapists often describe multiproblem patients as "therapy wise," meaning the patient can anticipate and counter the interventions of even the most skilled therapist. The number and magnitude of behavioral, cognitive, and emotional problems are a source of frustration for therapists. It is difficult to conceptualize a plan of action in therapy when, at any given point in time, the patient exhibits generalized failure in so many areas of functioning. Furthermore, the disruptive presence of chronic suicidal ideation, suicide attempting, and various other forms of self-destructive behavior can disrupt the continuity of treatment and can challenge the therapeutic relationship. Not surprisingly, existing research findings on the effectiveness of outpatient treatment reveal many gaps in our knowledge of how to treat such difficult patients. An unacceptably high rate of attrition from therapy (dropping out) has been found in most studies, and the best treatments available only seem to affect the frequency and lethality of suicide attempts while producing only limited effects on the more basic problems that fuel suicidal action. In essence, we would gladly trade all we know for all we do not know about the treatment of patients with suicidal lifestyles. With this caveat, we describe a set of treatment principles that may lead to a balanced and holistic approach to the treatment of repetitive suicidal behavior.

Suicide, Attempted Suicide, and Parasuicide

Much has been made in recent years of a possible distinction between patients who will ultimately commit suicide, patients who make suicide attempts, and parasuicidal patients. The term *parasuicide* was originally coined by Norman Kreitman (1977), a British researcher and clinician who noted that there seemed to be clinical differences between patients who are attracted to suicidal behavior for reasons other than the purpose of dying and those who are intent on dying, whether or not they succeed. In psychiatric parlance, the latter group is suicide attempters; the former group is parasuicide patients. Various speculations have ensued about how these groups might differ. For example, parasuicide patients are thought to be characterized by use of methods with low potential lethality, such as clearly sublethal drug overdosing, and action in a context in which discovery is highly likely. Conversely, suicide attempters have been described as using more lethal methods, even for drug overdosing, and as making efforts to elude detection. A major clinical milestone would be achieved if research were to isolate the characteristics that differentiate parasuicidal persons from those who attempt suicide. From the findings, clinicians would be able to identify patients most likely to engage in lethal forms of suicidal behavior.

Unfortunately, the utility of the distinction between parasuicide and attempted suicide has not been substantiated. For example, there is very little evidence that a patient's suicidal intent (i.e., intent to die, attempts to avoid discovery, and preplanning) is related to the medical severity of the attempts. High-intent patients may not be the same as the patients who end up in medical intensive care units. Clinical judgment has not been very accurate in separating these populations. With the exception of perceptions regarding the problem-solving value of suicide and the patient's ability to tolerate emotional pain, research has revealed very few differences between states of suicidality, even between patients who simply think about suicide and those who engage in some form of suicidal behavior.

In a study that included repetitious suicide attempters in an inpatient unit, we found subtle differences between low-intent and high-intent suicide attempters (Strosahl et al. 1992). Low-intent patients appear to be more influenced by hopelessness, depression, and low reasons for staying alive than do high-intent attempters. High-intent attempters report lower depression and hopelessness and more life-sustaining beliefs. The key issue to remember about this study is that these assessments were obtained after suicide attempts. High-intent attempters may have experienced more relief from anxiety secondary to their behavior and therefore reported less depression, less hopelessness, and a sense of being able to move on with their lives. In other words, the suicide attempt worked. Conversely, low-intent attempters may not have experienced the same degree of anxiety relief and problem resolution, perhaps because the attempt was seen as not serious; negative labeling occurred; and the problems either were not relieved or were made worse. Finally, recall that suicide intent itself, which is an assessment of the patient's self-reported intent to die, seems to have little to do with the probability of a completed suicide. In other words, these distinctions still do not reveal who is likely to die.

In a problem-solving framework, suicidal behavior is a method of managing distress. Many patients die because they were playing with fire. Their conscious intent to die might well have actually been ambivalent or even low. Conversely, high-intent patients discover that to commit suicide, everything has to work just right and a thousand things can go wrong. Bullets aimed at the heart have missed, hanging ropes have broken, and passersby have discovered and rescued many a near-dead individual. These factors lead to the following conclusion: Any form of suicidal behavior can be fatal. Attempting to label patients on the basis of lethality level not only is inaccurate but also can create major intervention errors.

Nevertheless, the concept of parasuicide has heavily influenced the British response to self-poisoning overdose (approximately 70% of suicide attempts) and has led to intervention techniques that have had positive outcome. In Great Britain, parasuicide has been defined as a syndrome requiring a distinct form of treatment. This definition has led to the creation of innovative and effective alternative treatment strategies, such as self-poisoning centers. In self-poisoning centers, patients are only medically assessed and stabilized; referral and discharge are immediate. Inpatient psychiatric hospitalization is only one of a variety of placement options. This approach has helped to make suicidal behavior a nonreinforcing event and to return the individual to the natural environment, where real-life problem solving can occur. Interestingly, the health care system in the United Kingdom has successfully used this low-intensity approach to repetitious self-poisoning and has violated some sacred precepts of American risk management in doing it.

A Functional Model of Repetitious Suicidal Behavior

From a functional perspective, multiproblem patients exhibit behavior patterns that are

- Pervasive: Maladaptive responses occur across a broad array of situations.
- Persistent: The responses are consistent over time.
- Resistant: The responses do not change despite negative consequences.
- Self-defeating: The responses defeat the patient's ultimate best interests.

To work effectively with the repetitiously suicidal patient, it is important that you place less emphasis on the patient's diagnostic label (a structural concept) and place more emphasis on the functions that support the maintenance of unworkable patterns of behavior. To this end, it will be useful to briefly examine these four concepts in more detail.

Pervasiveness of Maladaptive Behavior

Patients do not experience pervasive life difficulties by being dysfunctional in discrete and limited situations. Their behavior has to be ineffective across a broad range of situations. Pervasive dysfunctional responses can be the result of generalized rule-governed responses. Rule-governed behavior is a core concept of relational frame theory, a behavioral analytic account of the functional properties of human language and thought. A rule-governed behavior is one that is the result of arbitrarily derived relationships generated by basic language functions; in effect, it is behavior that is driven by "rules" that the patient has acquired. The problem is that rule-governed responses generalize rapidly because of the very properties of language and thought that make humans so adaptive. Thus a rule-governed response might work very well in one situation but might be ineffective in a second situation that shares only a fraction of the same attributes as the first situation. Even so, the rule-governed response tends to generalize to the second situation. In functional terms, the patient does not make appropriate discriminations between situations that share some, but not many, overlapping attributes. This lack of discrimination results in a narrowing of responses in the patient's coping hierarchy. For example, any interpersonal conflict involving anger, no matter what the anger is about, whom it involves or how serious it is, elicits the same response from the patient. In essence, the patient is treating every situation using the same rule rather than being responsive and flexible to the features of each situation. One of our patients once remarked in the course of therapy, "I don't do anger." This type of response narrowing is possible only in humans and reflects the dark side of human language and thought.

Another potential contributor to pervasive behavior is the absence of skills in key life areas (e.g., personal problem solving, tolerance for distress, and interpersonal effectiveness). Thus the patient is left with a narrow set of coping responses that will be used across a broad range of life situations. Quite literally, the patient emits the same behavioral response in qualitatively different situations because the patient only has one response to give. The genesis of this problem may be found in the childhood and adolescent histories of repetitiously suicidal patients. Study findings suggest these people tend to have a high incidence of childhood trauma, including physical and sexual abuse. In addition, these patients tend to come from dysfunctional settings involving problems such as parental mental illness, drug addiction, alcoholism, and domestic assault. Additional studies suggest that trauma is strongly related to defects in memory encoding and retrieval. Some of these recall deficits appear to represent a very basic form of emotional avoidance. By not being able to recall past events specifically, the patient also avoids the emotional content associated with events. The problem is that a person who cannot recall the past with enough specificity will not be able to learn new responses quickly.

A second mechanism of action is that dysfunctional environments model inappropriate coping and problem-solving skills for children and adolescents. These responses are then integrated into the child's repertoire. In essence, ineffective, dysfunctional parents tend to turn out ineffective, dysfunctional children. In the treatment of suicidal patients, it is important to look for and remedy specific skill deficits that may be contributing to the patient's problematic behavior. For example, studies have shown that multiproblem patients lack physiological control skills (knowing how to relieve arousal), personal problem-solving skills, goal-setting and self-directed change skills, and both social and assertion skills, to name but a few.

Persistence of Dysfunctional Behavior

A seminal attribute of multiproblem behavior patterns is that they can occur for years, despite consistent negative social reinforcement and pressure to change exerted by the verbal community. Two major mechanisms account for the durability of these problematic behaviors. One is that the behavior "works" in the sense that it generates internal and external reinforcements. Repetitiously suicidal patients use suicidal and self-destructive behavior to control affective arousal and solve problems in the environment. We discuss this concept at length later (see Three Therapy Process Issues With the Repetitiously Suicidal Patient), but from a reinforcement perspective, there is good reason to believe that suicidal and self-destructive behavior generates powerful and immediate reinforcements that override the patient's ability to change behavior based on longer-term consequences.

A second mechanism is related to the generalization of rule-governed responses over time, not just across situations. Much the same way we can read a Shakespeare play written 400 years ago and generate all of the thoughts and emotions of the key characters, a patient can carry a set of rule-governed behaviors over a lifetime. Rule-governed behavior generalizes rapidly and can become embedded in so many frames of reference that it is almost impossible to extinguish. At a point, the dysfunctional response is almost automatic and beneath the level of self-awareness. Because of these characteristics, it is important to use self-observation, mindfulness, and simple awareness strategies with suicidal patients. If it is not observed from the position of being an observer, rule-governed thinking is very difficult to detect.

Another important feature of rule-governed behavior is that it is strongly influenced by other language-based processes. One clinically significant process is *augmentation.* Augmentation occurs when a positive conceptualized future reward is used to strengthen adherence to a present rule. One of us (K.S.) worked with a suicidal patient who used this augmental technique to strengthen her suicidal responses: "I want my mother to suffer for all the damage she did to me." The conceptualized future of her mother suffering increases the dominance of the patient's rule-governed response (emotional avoidance and resulting suicidal behavior). Every time she makes a suicide attempt, the patient not only is following her internally generated rule about how to deal with suffering but also experiences the augmentation of her mother suffering for her sins. Research in relational frame theory shows that augmentation can drive behavior that produces unequivocally negative results.

Resistance to Change

Resistance means that the dysfunctional behavior pattern is not changing, despite negative results and pressure from self or others to adopt new behavior patterns. This characteristic of multiproblem patients is extremely challenging for therapists. The patient's life is falling apart. The patient is in great emotional pain. Why can't (or won't) the patient change problematic behaviors?

The most toxic effect of rule-governed behavior is that it is not responsive to shifting contingencies. In other words, once a rule-governed response is formed, it overrides the consequences of the behaviors it generates. What multiproblem patients seem to lack is a certain type of psychological flexibility. They do not seem to learn new responses on the basis of the results of old responses. In other words, they do not exhibit behaviors shaped by contingencies (results). Contingency-shaped behavior is a response that works in the specific context in which it is emitted. If you go outside in a T-shirt when the temperature is −20°F, you will rapidly develop a new behavior linked to going outside. It is called "putting your warmest coat on." If, however, you walk outside in your warmest coat and the temperature is 100°F, you will rapidly develop a new rule called "wear your lightest shirt outside." Instead of figuratively changing garments as a result of contact with the temperature, a multi-problem patient may say, "Listen, my mother taught me to wear my T-shirt, and that's what I'm going to do. It's unfair that the temperature changes like this. Other people don't have to deal with this. This symbolizes how life victimizes me."

Flexible, effective human responding requires that we stay in touch with the contingencies of each particular situation and adapt our behavior accordingly. Multiproblem patients, however, live in a cognitive world that is overrun with simple and inflexible rules, a world in which following the rules means everything. In short, if a rule states that you should engage in behavior X, then the most important thing to do is do behavior X. There is no particular importance attached to determining whether behavior X works in this specific context.

What types of rule-governed responses can exercise this dominance over direct experience? The following are examples of what you might hear clinically:

I just need to gain control over the way I'm feeling.

Painful feelings are bad for you; you must eliminate them.

The goal of healthy living is to be relatively free of emotional pain.

I will not allow myself to have feeling X because healthy people don't have it.

These samples demonstrate an important quality of rule-governed responses. The highly generalized rules are strongly shaped by the culture in which we live. Most of us have come into contact with these rules, and to some degree, we can see them as rules we might or might not follow. A multiproblem patient, however, sees not rules but mandates for how life is to be lived. This matter is not one of logic; it is a matter of a rule's gaining dominance over direct experience. Because it is more important to follow the rule than observe how the resulting behavior worked, a likely explanation for failure in a situation is, "I don't have what it takes to follow that rule. I need more (confidence, support from others, intelligence, willpower) or less (depression, anxiety, self-loathing, anger) and then the rule will work." Work with a repetitiously suicidal patient always involves pointing out rules and seeing them as rules. To free himself or herself from the hegemony of rule following, the patient first needs to observe these rules as inflexible, self-defeating structures.

Behavior That Is Self-Defeating

What do we mean by the term "self-defeating"? Simply put, self-defeating behaviors are responses that do not work in a given context. These responses might work in another context, but they are not adaptive in the present one. What does "working" mean? It means producing responses that address a situation in a way that promotes the person's sense of vitality, purpose, and meaning. When we see chronically dysfunctional patients in therapy, a singular impression is that they are literally and figuratively having the life squeezed out of them. They not only are persistently suicidal but also seem psychologically dead. If you were to ask, "What would you be doing in your life if you weren't stewing around in your suicidal thoughts and behavior all the time?" the answer would probably be, "I don't know." This destination is eventually reached by those engaged in excessive, ineffective rule following. Life is about following the rules, not about enjoying being alive. Rather than responding to life's challenges from a position of personal values and goals, the patient is simply following rules. With patients who have been suicidal for years, it is not unusual to get the sense that there are no values driving the patient's behavior. Because behavior is always being driven by something, this assessment is not really true, but it speaks volumes about the life-suppressing quality of rule-governed behavior.

The trap our patients are in is that it is not possible to succeed at following the rules because the events specified in them are not amenable to direct manipulation, control, or elimination. For someone who has chronic problems with depressive symptoms, the goal is not to use willpower to suppress the symptoms. The person's goal is to accept that he or she has symptoms and move on with his or her life. Paradoxically, when negative private experiences are suppressed or avoided, they actually gain more dominance. The rule-governed response becomes self-amplifying, not because it works but because it does not. The more the patient tries to suppress the depression, the more depressed he or she becomes. The rule-governed response is called up more and more frequently. Because rule-governed responding is not sensitive to contingencies, the patient is left to look for explanations for failure that do not include challenging the general workability of the rule. It is not unusual to hear multiproblem patients emphatically state (as a fact) that other people can control their depression, anxiety, flashbacks, and so on. Thus the patient 1) is not trying hard enough, 2) lacks the necessary willpower or character to make a change, or 3) is inadequate and inept. At the far end of this process, the suicidal lifestyle, the self-amplifying quality of emotional control, avoidance, and suppression sweep over the patient's life space like a tidal wave. The human being is buried under a wall of water, nowhere to be found. In therapy with repetitiously suicidal patients, it is important to look for and "wake up" the person being buried alive by his or her rules.

See the World Your Repetitiously Suicidal Patient Sees

Our clinical experience suggests that therapists find it difficult to relate to chronically suicidal, multiproblem patients. Therapists have trouble looking on the patient with the same compassion, empathy, and understanding available for more functional clients. Perhaps this difficulty is due to discomfort with suicidal behavior, fear of litigation, or fear of being ineffective. Whatever the reason, it is difficult to be effective with a patient if there is no grasp of the patient's outlook on life. If that context cannot be created in therapy, the context that will be used is the therapist's outlook. It is important for the therapist to bring an outlook into the room, but it cannot be the dominant outlook. The dominant outlook is the patient's perspective on how the world seems to be working. Therapists who do well with such patients are able to see the world through the eyes of the patient and can get in touch with the private logic the person uses to explain pervasive patterns of unworkable behavior.

The repetitiously suicidal patient often has a multitude of psychological deficits associated with suicidal behavior. The deficits may not be qualitatively different from those of the person who experiences a single suicidal crisis only. What makes the repetitious patient difficult to treat is the manner in which these multiple deficits interact negatively with both a worldview and a self-view to produce a suicidal lifestyle. Multiproblem, repetitiously suicidal individuals often have a dysfunctional family background characterized by adverse events, sexual and physical abuse, neglect, parental addiction or alcoholism, parental abandonment, or a combination of these problems. Many of these patients have matured in a trauma-filled environment that has provided scarce opportunities for learning the necessary skills for surviving and thriving in the real world. Table 6–1 lists some of the more common beliefs about self and the world that can form the basis of a multiproblem patient's adaptation to the demands of life.

As Table 6–1 shows, very little is elegant about the day-to-day reality of multiproblem patients. Their lives are characterized by emotional pain, a constant struggle to meet the demands of living, and interpersonal conflict or isolation. In a world producing continuous discomfort, the rule of survival is simple. If something helps lessen the pain of a situation, it is used again and again without regard to long-term consequences, which are for people who *have* a future. With adherence to this simple rule, there are few problem-solving behaviors that work as quickly and as effectively as suicidal behavior. Suicidal behavior relieves pent-up frustration and anxiety, creates an environment oriented toward providing attention and caring, and helps the individual escape from what is often a painful and hopeless living situation. Make no mistake about it: Suicidal behavior is a very effective problem-solving behavior if one is willing to risk possible (even if considered unlikely) death and is willing to ignore long-term consequences. The better you can understand this world as the therapist, the more comfortable you will be in addressing the patient's struggles.

A Basic Treatment Approach

We have analyzed repetitive suicidal behavior from both the functional and the behavioral points of view. We are working with patients who engage in the same unworkable behavior over and over again. They do it because of the dominance of rule-governed thought and a lack of specific skills. This behavior suggests a treatment approach designed to undermine the use of high-risk emotional avoidance behaviors to get the patient in contact with the costs of rule following, to encourage the development of responses that are contingency governed, and to begin building patterns of committed action based in personal values. Table 6–2 presents a synthesis of the phases of this treatment approach along with clinical targets. The following are the key themes to which you need to attend.

Table 6–1.   World- and self-related beliefs of the multiproblem patient

I. Beliefs about the world

   A. The more important it is, the less likely it is to happen.
   B. When you expect good things, bad things will happen.
   C. Negative thoughts and feelings are destructive.
   D. Life cannot proceed in the presence of suffering.
   E. The only way to change is just decide to be different.
   F. Make a mistake and you will be punished for it.
   G. The goal with suffering is to get rid of it.
   H. Life is basically unpredictable and unfair.
   I. Do unto others before they do unto you.

II. Beliefs about self

   A. I am flawed in a basic way.
   B. I don't deserve to be happy.
   C. If I can't do it well, I won't do it at all.
   D. I must understand why I am the way I am or I can't be different.
   E. I will end up killing myself.
   F. I don't fit in.
   G. I am permanently damaged by my past.
   H. If I let my emotions go, I will go crazy.
   I. Killing myself is the easiest way out.

Phase One: Create a Humanizing Clinical Foothold

There are a number of priorities when you first start working with a repetitiously suicidal patient. One of the most important priorities is to create motivation in the patient to stay in therapy long enough for some benefit to occur. The rate of attrition from treatment among these patients is very high, and no therapy works when the patient is not attending sessions. Both therapist and client variables must be controlled. On the therapist side, you must repeatedly validate the patient's sense of emotional desperation and avoid using pathological explanations to frame the patient's behavior. You should emphasize the problem-solving nature of suicidal behavior—that it is one legitimate way of attacking the problem of human suffering. If suicidal behavior occurs during this phase (and it usually does), reframe the behavior as a

Table 6–2.   An outpatient treatment model for the repetitiously suicidal patient

Phase one: Establish a humanizing clinical framework

- Reframe the function of the behavior.
- Neutralize the reinforcements for engaging in suicidal behavior.
- Study rather than judge the behavior.
- Emphasize "response ability" rather than blame.
- Use suicidal crises as opportunities for exploring two alternatives: acceptance (willingness) and control (struggle).
- Connect the patient with the cost of emotional avoidance in valued life goals.
- Develop a crisis and case management framework.

Phase two: Attack both the rationale for and workability of suicidal behavior

- Get patient to invest in the "story."
- Destabilize confidence in the story.
- Institute workability as the yardstick.
- Help patient disengage from rational, but futile, emotional control rules.
- Encourage stopping what does not work before looking for what does work.

Phase three: Substitute acceptance and willingness for emotional control

- Study relationship of willingness, suffering, and workability.
- Reframe suicidal behavior as a choice, not a decision.
- Find small ways to practice willingness.
- Use experiential exercises and mindfulness to teach patient to detach from unworkable rules.

Phase four: Develop expanding patterns of committed action

- Help patient clarify valued ends in basic sectors of living (values clarification).
- Help patient develop value-based goals.
- Emphasize small committed actions and accumulating positives.
- Use acceptance to sustain movement through psychological barriers.
- Relate sense of victimization, responsibility, and blame with forgiveness.
- Emphasize committed action as a process, not an outcome.

choice between making room for negative events and eliminating them. We begin using self-monitoring diaries early in treatment to teach the patient self-observation skills. At all times, you must avoid getting into showdowns over suicidal behavior. You must avoid strategies such as moralizing about suicide, lecturing the patient, and taking an overly proscriptive approach. This phase is oriented toward forming a collaborative therapeutic relationship, creating a credible therapeutic model of suicidal behavior, and helping the patient to see the scope and nature of the real problem.

On the client side, you want to get the patient in touch with the cost of chronic suicidal behavior. The intent of questions such as, Tell me, have your problems with suicidality affected other goals you have in life? Were there things you dreamed of doing in life that seem far out of reach now? In terms of your personal values, how does suicidal behavior fit in? and Is it consistent with what you want to be about as a human being? is to get the patient thinking about the relationship between personal values and a suicidal lifestyle. The patient ultimately has to determine that suicidal behavior is not working, even though the rule-governed response class (suicidal behavior/emotional avoidance) will still exist. This approach will help create openness to contingency-shaped responding. At the early stage of treatment, getting in touch with the cost is also a motivational enhancement strategy.

The final goal of the first phase is to establish a sound crisis and case management framework. A sound crisis and case management framework is designed to neutralize to the extent possible the external and internal reinforcements of suicidal behavior. This framework also establishes a set of agreements about how the patient and the therapist will deal with recurrent suicidal crises. We discuss this concept later (see The Moment of Truth: The First Crisis in Treatment). In addition, Chapter 7 ("Managing Suicidal Emergencies") contains information you can use to establish a behaviorally based crisis and case management framework.

Phase Two: Attack the Rationale for, and the Workability of, Suicidal Behavior

An important concept in this treatment approach is to undermine the patient's confidence in his or her "story." The story is the patient's set of verbally articulated reasons for using suicidal behavior and the patient's rationale for seeing this behavior as an effective device. The story often contains important clues to the presence of rule-governed responses. The patient may tell you a tale of woe that goes back to childhood abuse, broken relationships, unloving parents, or failed life goals. Somewhere in the patient's story, you will begin to encounter certain assumptions the patient has about how he or she came to such suffering and why suicidal behavior is a necessary and justifiable response. The rationale for suicidal behavior usually is that the patient cannot or will not tolerate a particular type of negative private event (flashbacks, anger, or feelings that are difficult to tolerate). There is a structural similarity in most stories because they originate in language and culture. In other words, the patient will use the story to explain the presence of chronic suicidal behavior as well as to justify it. Do not challenge the story in terms of its logic; just get a sense of how the various elements of the story pull together to rationalize the behavior. Rule-governed responses function in this manner in practice. A patient's life can be in total disarray, and yet the story can provide good reasons for the disarray.

The way to effectively maneuver in the context of the patient's story is to use the concept of workability. *Workability* means that the behavior is promoting the patient's sense of vitality, purpose, and meaning. This concept is not something to argue about with the patient. After all, it is not your life that is being lived here, and the patient may have some very different ideas about what constitutes a workable life. For the most part, the workability question goes something like this: "So, as I understand it, you have problem X, then feeling Y, and then you engage in behavior Z as a response to problem X and feeling Y. How is behavior Z working in the sense of promoting your sense of being a valuing person with life purpose and meaning?" Then you let the patient answer the question. We use this question over and over again in all sorts of clinical moments. It is a very effective way to get "unhooked" from a negative therapeutic interaction. We give you a chance to practice your responses to this type of event in the Dealing With Downers exercise.

Eventually you will begin to put a name to the problem that is confounding the patient. A major observation in acceptance and commitment therapy is, "Gain control of your feelings, lose control of your life." Repetitiously suicidal patients are the walking embodiment of this theme. Their entire lives are out of control because they insist on emotional control. These patients avoid things they cannot control. At this point in treatment, it is important to begin calling out this change agenda. You can deconstruct instances of suicidal behavior from exactly this perspective. Again, it is not something to argue about with the patient. You are not playing a game in which you are trying to be right and showing the patient to be wrong. Simply note in a nonjudgmental way that there seems to be a similarity over time and situations in the methods the patient is using to respond to events.

Phase Three: Substitute Acceptance and Willingness for Emotional Control

If the patient sees emotional control as unworkable, it is time to pose an alternative. That alternative is to accept your thoughts, feelings, sensations, and memories and do what needs to be done to promote a valued, purposeful life. There are two important concepts in this phase. One is that willingness to be negative to an event is a choice and action specific to each life situation. There is a strong relationship between being unwilling to experience things directly and emotional suffering. The experience of an unwanted feeling, a feeling one is struggling to avoid, is truly traumatic. An unwanted feeling experienced directly, without struggle, is simply painful. Pain is a natural component of human existence. It is not toxic in itself. Human organisms are built to feel what they feel, think what they think, and remember what they remember. The destructive component is the avoidance behaviors that develop from following rules that suggest direct human experience is dangerous, toxic, or diminishing. You can help the patient begin to appreciate this paradox by looking situation by situation at the relationship between levels of willingness, levels of suffering, and life workability. The other thing to realize is you do not get willingness forever, like a trophy hanging on the wall. Willingness and acceptance are moment-to-moment events. Sometimes we are willing and accepting; other times we are not. You do not want the patient to co-opt this idea into a rigid rule-following system, so that is read, "My problem is that I was abused as a child, and I just don't have enough willingness. What you are telling me is that if I was just more willing to have pain, then my pain would be less." Your answer is "Yes, willingness means showing up for whatever is there and allowing it to be whatever it will become, without struggle or defense."

The second theme in this phase is that you must help your patient learn what the detached mode looks and feels like. It is important to use various experiential exercises, metaphors, and mindfulness tactics within each session. You want to teach the patient that there is a position from which the content of living is seen for what it is, not what it advertises it to be. In acceptance and commitment therapy, this process is called *defusion*. Defusion strategies help the patient separate self from the contents of being alive. Consult the Selected Readings for the myriad strategies used in this regard. Another important aspect of detachment is that it allows the person to engage in a contingency-shaped response. The patient can now ask, "If I'm not going to run from the situation, how will I respond to it?" The answer varies from situation to situation, but a general rule might be, "Do what works to promote your sense of humanness." At this stage a patient may need help in learning specific skills such as personal problem solving, assertion, social skills, and conflict resolution. Begin one or more of these traditional skills-training interventions as soon as your patient understands that these skills are to be put in the service of approach and resolution, not avoidance and self-annihilation.

Phase Four: Develop Expanding Patterns of Committed Action

As treatment progresses, you will encounter the following basic question: "If your life is not going to be about being suicidal all the time, what is it going to be about?" Your goal is to help the patient find the answer to this question. One of our favorite ways of approaching this issue is to ask, "What do you want your life to stand for? Is suicidal behavior and self-mutilation consistent with that?" We are trying to wake up the human being and bring out the best in him or her. Standing for something in life is very important, because it drives behavior and legitimizes the pain and suffering that are part and parcel of participating in life. We are not teaching the patient to accept painful material simply for the sake of acceptance. That would be sadistic. Rather, the importance of acceptance is that it allows the patient to set aside barriers to committed action. Instead of using anger as a reason not to perform in a valued way, the patient can make room for anger and behave in a way that is consistent with his or her values as a human being. Valuing is presented as a free human act. The patient gets to choose how to respond, because values are not certainties—they are just an assumptive part of human existence. Valued and committed action also frees the patient from the hegemony of rule-governed behavior. This type of action increases the likelihood that the patient's behavior can be contingency shaped rather than rule governed.

In therapy, you can initiate limited-scale committed action. There is a quality to committed action that is not measured by the size or importance of the act but by the freedom of the act. Hence, it is fine to start small and establish an atmosphere of success. Over time, your patient will begin to spontaneously initiate valued actions in all sorts of situations.

One thing to watch for at this point is the reappearance of the patient's story in an insidious form. After all, if the story is one of abuse, neglect, and lack of love leading to a broken human being, what is the significance of that same person's ending up with a vital, purposeful life? It could mean that the alleged perpetrator was not wrong and might be let off the hook of blame. We have seen more than one patient who, when confronted with the likelihood of a meaningful life, relapsed into serious suicidality. Your patients are attached to their stories. Freud was right about that—sometimes the old ruins tremble. Normally, as the patient begins to show more psychological flexibility, it is important to talk about how past pain and trauma, blame and responsibility may interfere with choosing committed action. A typical question we might ask is, Who would be let off the hook of blame if you were to get better and lead a good life? It is useful to talk about forgiveness in this context, not as an act toward the perpetrator but as an act toward the self. That is what the word *forgiveness* means in its Latin root—literally, to give oneself the grace that came before. The task is not about forgetting bad acts or liking the people who performed them, it is about giving oneself permission to move on.

Three Therapy Process Issues With the Repetitiously Suicidal Patient

For some individuals and in some situations, a clinician can cause a patient to perform in more adaptive ways by the exercise of personal authority. As an expert, you state what needs to be done, and your patient follows this advice. You are in a professional role, that of a healer, your suggestions are sound, and your motive is to be helpful. The individual seeking your help does what you say. Some individuals, however, do not respond to authority in this manner. They push the issue of who has control in the patient-clinician interaction. These patients may be labeled as having personality disorders; they are uncooperative because they have not accepted your treatment. If treatment becomes stalled at this point, you can end up feeling defeated, powerless, and angry. These negative reactions can sometimes be transferred onto your patient in the form of pejorative labels, such as *borderline trait, manipulative, insincere, oppositional,* and *defiant.*

Given the dynamic in caring for a repetitiously suicidal patient, it is important to note that there are many potential sources of polarization between you and the patient. *The most initially troublesome is usually the acceptability or unacceptability of using self-destructive behavior to solve problems.* Most people are taught to regulate their behavior primarily around an evaluation of long-term consequences. The clinician, likely being one of these people, has difficulty accepting the notion that someone will knowingly engage in repetitious suicidal behavior. Dangerously, the clinician may attribute malevolent intentions to the patient (i.e., the patient is deliberately doing bad things).

A second polarity relates to differences in both the perception of suffering and what to do about it. You may come from a world in which people are taught to endure their suffering while finding constructive ways to regulate and solve problems. Your patient often comes from a world that is strictly focused on getting rid of suffering. Your patient can be in the unenviable position of being unwilling to accept emotional pain while being told that the outside world does not accept the only available solution for getting rid of that pain.

A third polarity involves trying to get better versus trying to get by. You will usually emphasize that improvement is possible, whereas your patient's experience may be that trying to improve things does not work. Attempts at improvement may have backfired, especially if your patient comes from a dysfunctional family or if a dysfunctional support network is present. Some therapists tend to link emotional validation and support to evidence that their patient is doing something constructive about problems. This attitude makes it difficult to provide attention and caring in the face of destructive solutions for pain and suffering. The patient wants to be cared for even though the life plan is just to get by. Consequently, the actions in which the patient is most likely to engage to solve problems (e.g., suicidal behavior) are also the most likely to draw negative reactions from the therapist and therefore put the issue of the therapist's ability to care for the patient on the table.

In addition to these sources of polarization, some clinicians have unreasonable rescue and power fantasies that become activated in a showdown motif: Can the therapist stop the patient from using self-destructive behavior? The impasse that results over this issue can be fatal for treatment. It can produce increased episodes of suicidal behavior, lack of compliance with treatment, resistance interpretations, therapy dropout, and therapist "dumps" into different layers of the treatment system. Both the clinician and the patient can spend a great deal of energy on feeling frustrated, angry, and misunderstood. In the uncontained case, the patient may begin to use suicidal behavior in an attempt to solve the impasse with the clinician, just as the patient would use the same problem-solving approach in the natural world.

Reconciling Opposites With the Repetitious Patient

To reach the chronically suicidal patient, you must realize that the more pressure you apply to eliminating suicidal behavior, the more intractable suicidal behavior may become. The process that occurs between the push of the clinician and the push back of the patient needs to be harnessed for constructive purposes. Following the principle that the surest way to avoid loss in a tug-of-war is to drop the rope, this treatment approach focuses on techniques that allow you to drop negative polarities while making strategic use of polarizing processes.

Allow Your Patient "to Be"

From the viewpoint of acceptance and commitment therapy, your patient is not broken, only trapped in an unworkable change agenda. This strategy honors the fact that your patient is "response able," literally meaning able to engage in valued actions no matter how severe and intractable the situation. It is important to differentiate between being response able (in Old English, this term literally meant to be alive, not dead) and "responsible." The latter term suggests a right and wrong aspect to a behavior and thus promotes blaming in therapy. The concept of being response able acknowledges that each of us has the ability to choose a response to any given situation. The ability to choose is what dignifies the client's actions. The critical strategy in this regard is to give your patient room to make choices, even choices that are based on old and unhealthful behaviors. The fact is, your patient can be unhealthy despite your best efforts, so allow the patient "to be." For example, it is useful to preempt the issue of stopping suicidal behavior by predicting that it may occur during treatment. Although you need to be clear about related case management and crisis procedures, the important message is that a recurrence of suicidal behavior is not going to result in a power struggle. *If it happens, it happens. We will learn from it, and treatment will proceed.*

Look for and reinforce positive elements in whatever your patient has done. Rather than criticizing a patient who has just overdosed, focus on any and all positive thoughts and actions that occurred during the suicidal episode. Search for problem-solving behaviors that occurred before the drug overdose and strongly praise your patient for trying those things. For example, look for attempts to contact others for help, for maneuvers to reduce emotional distress, and for any techniques your patient may have used to get through the difficult period. Praise any effort to steer the episode toward more effective problem solving. For example, if your patient did not attempt to contact other people but thought of doing so, praise the thought. These techniques create an acceptance of suicidal behavior as a form of problem solving, an acknowledgment that your patient is struggling and trying his or her best, and an atmosphere that always encourages other ways to look at difficulties.

Steal the Point of Resistance

Stealing the point of resistance is one of many strategies you should use to undercut the evaluative, black-and-white thinking style that is so pervasive among multiproblem patients. This strategy involves your being the first to find the limitation of any nonsuicidal problem-solving strategy. For example, in a dialogue with your patient about a way to solve a particular problem, occasionally play the devil's advocate by stating all the reasons suicidal behavior would work better than the new alternative. It is important to develop a sense of timing with this intervention. Look for moments when your patient seems to be losing a problem-solving focus and begins making superficial and poorly thought through comments about needing to find other ways to solve difficulties. Intervene by pointing out that suicidal behavior has been far too important to be whisked away in this manner. In general, anticipate a possible point of polarity and occupy the negative pole, so that your patient can either agree with you or take the positive pole in an attempt to maintain polarity. This technique is based on the assumption that the chronically suicidal patient is a disillusioned optimist—that is, the patient really wants to believe that things can be changed for the better but has had so many disconfirming experiences that a *fear develops about being hopeful.* When given the opportunity, the suicidal patient may unexpectedly occupy the optimistic pole and may even express some disbelief or confusion about your apparent pessimism. Ironically, when you take the apparently negative, pessimistic position, your patient often feels understood and validated. The act of embodying your patient's sense of frustration and negativism is an act of empathy. The fact that there is an ever-present potential for suicidal behavior can make you feel constantly obligated to challenge the patient's negative worldviews. Remember that being willing to identify with your patient's negative worldview can create a new context in which to discuss persistent suicidal ideation and behavior.

Sympathize With Suicidal Impulses

Sympathizing with suicidal impulses is a technique designed to validate emotional pain while reframing what are often experienced as uncontrollable suicidal impulses. When your patient is feeling suicidal, make a concerted effort to identify all of the patient's problems and then state that many individuals would consider suicide if faced with such a multitude of difficulties. Acknowledging that there is a universal connection between feeling frustrated and blocked and considering suicide is a way of slipping the problem-solving notion in the back door. In other words, suicidal behavior is moved off center when you empathize with your patient's sense of emotional pain and frustration while at the same time linking repetitious suicidal behavior and unsolved problems. Many difficulties can mean suicidal behavior for almost anyone. Let your patient know that he or she is not alone in this feeling and that the need to face suicidality and get on with life can arise in all of us and at any time. A motto you need in working with this type of patient is "We are in this stew together."

Make Suicidal Impulses an *It*

One of the defining features of repetitious suicidal patients is the pervasiveness of intense suicidal ideation and suicidal impulses. In other words, the patient is completely fused with these private events. When these events occur (and they do with alarming frequency), the patient responds by attaching to the thought or urge, such that there is no free space between the patient and the suicidal event. Put in simple parlance, your patient is not having suicidal urges, the suicidal urges are having the patient. One of the most effective ways to help the patient defuse from destructive impulses is to develop the capacity to comment about you as a person having these impulses and to move out of your participant role and into an observer role. A good image to suggest is this: "Put parentheses around yourself in this suicidal situation. Now step outside the parentheses and look at that person dealing with that problem. Describe what you see." The capacity to use this imagery transforms the functions of the suicidal thought or urge from an *I am* event (meaning that a behavioral intention will be formed) to an *it,* an entity to be observed, commented on, and accepted for what it is (just a thought). As an *it*, the suicidal thought loses the aura of overwhelming force to which your patient must succumb.

When your patient reaches the point of stepping outside the situation at the moment he or she is in it, then a truly significant advance will have been made. Questions such as, What do your suicidal thoughts have to say about trying something new in this situation? help your patient externalize and encapsulate suicidal impulses. By giving the thoughts entity or *it* status, these impulses become endowed through linguistic association with their own motives. You can then place these motivations at odds with something your patient really wants, for example, Do you think your suicidal impulses are really going to stand for your having a good time this weekend? What do you think they'll do to ruin it for you? The implicit goal of these maneuvers is to separate the patient from the suicidal impulses and to create a greater contrast between what the patient thinks and what the patient is. The capacity to extract the *self* out of suffering is a prerequisite for any acceptance.

Suicidal Feelings Are Your Friends

The chronically suicidal patient comes to rely on feeling suicidal as a way of gaining reassurance. Even though such feelings are experienced as uncontrollable and alien at one level, at another basic level they are familiar, predictable experiences in an otherwise chaotic world. If all else fails to create meaning, the patient can always fall back on being suicidal (e.g., "Thoughts of suicide have gotten me through many a bad night."). It is important to honor this relationship between your patient and suicidal impulses. Point out that gaining reassurance is an extremely vital human need and that nothing in therapy is designed to break that important bond. For a patient who has been repeatedly stigmatized for having such feelings, having the reassuring function of suicidal thoughts acknowledged and protected can be a major step toward viewing these experiences in a different context.

The ultimate behavioral goal of these reconciling strategies is to create a therapeutic moment in which your patient does a double take. This reaction indicates that your patient has just run into a piece of information outside of his or her operational frame of reference. When your patient has to form a new, more accepting context for relating to key issues, the pressure to engage in suicidal behavior is likely to diminish. This progress means not that existing skill deficits have been remedied but that the situation has become more amenable to development of other ways of adapting to circumstances. It is very difficult to promote behavioral change in the face of unacceptable suicidal impulses and the consequent frequent self-destructive behavior. Change becomes easier as the impulses become friendlier, more amenable, and more open to being dealt with.

Dealing With Downers

Working with the repetitiously suicidal patient is made difficult by the recurrence of communications that put you in a bind: Any response you think of seems likely to make things worse. Most patients have been conditioned to expect failure and interpersonal disappointment, so their immediate reaction to almost any attempt to help is to downplay the sincerity or the competency of the helper. Your patient may tend to cling tenaciously to suicidality as if it were a security blanket, appearing so sensitized to failure and rejection that the encouragement to even experiment with alternative problem solving seems too risky. The recurrence of situations that seem set up for rejection can be traced to the ongoing influence of the polarities discussed earlier in Three Therapy Process Issues With the Repetitiously Suicidal Patient. Although it is impossible to anticipate every variation on these themes, the overall success of treatment is in large part determined by the consistency and quality of your responses.

The Dealing With Downers exercise in Table 6–3 is designed to allow you to experiment with likely responses to common conundrums that are presented by suicidal patients. The first part of the exercise lists patient statements. Your job is to generate a response that validates the patient's reality while eschewing a confrontation or disappointment. The second part contains sample responses that meet the criteria of being consistent, nonjudgmental, and confirming of the patient. Do not look at them until you have completed the exercise. As you complete the exercise, imagine that you are face to face with a suicidal patient. Also, keep in mind the following principles:

1. Beware of overly judgmental or defensive responses. Try to see your patient's communication as a statement about a certain view of the world, not as a criticism of your competence.
2. Find a way to validate the emotionally painful part of the communication in a way that is sincere and honest.
3. Find a way to separate the thought, feeling, or action that is being described from the person having these experiences.

Table 6–3. Dealing With Downers exercise: patient statements and therapist sample responses

Patient statements

A. I really do want to die.

B. Everything is fine; I don't need to do anything.

C. It doesn't matter anyway.

D. Why don't you focus your time on helping someone who has a chance?

E. It's just too hard to do.

F. What would you do if you felt like I do?

G. I don't want to talk about it. It's stupid.

H. It will take forever to change.

I. I don't care one way or the other.

J. It would be nice if it were just all over.

K. That's baloney. [In response to your statement of caring.]

L. Nothing is working. Nothing is working. It just doesn't help.

M. There is only one way to feel better.

N. I don't know what I feel. Why do you keep asking?

O. This therapy isn't working. I don't feel any better than when we started.

P. I have pills, and I'm going to use them.

Q. [Via telephone call at 3:00 A.M.]: I just want you to know that you are a very nice person. Whatever I do, I don't want you to take it personally.

Therapist sample responses

A. *It sounds like you've got a lot of problems, and, at least for now, you think suicide would solve them. If you did kill yourself, what thoughts or feelings would you be getting out from under that right now you just can't accept?*

B. [If context is anger]: *It sounds like you are feeling fairly frustrated.* [If context is denial]: *There is a lot going on in your life, and we both know there is much to be done. Maybe this is one of those times when you need to block everything out. How has blocking things out like this worked in the past?*

C. *It sounds like what you've been doing to cope with this situation isn't working. Let's take a look at what those strategies have been and how they have and haven't worked.*

D. [If question is based on hopelessness or worthlessness]: *I am. You do have a chance.* [If question is in the context of testing the therapist and can be rephrased as, "Do you care about me?"]: *Regardless of what you think about your situation, I do care about the way it works out. I think we can work together and make things better for you.*

E. *Looking at change from a certain point of view can sure make it seem that way. Change is not easy for anyone, especially if it involves accepting painful realities.*

Table 6–3.   Dealing With Downers exercise: patient statements and therapist sample responses *(continued)*

F.   *I might well think about killing myself, and I hope I would be as smart as you were and get some help.*

G.   *That's cool. Just talking about things like this isn't the same as doing things differently in your life. If you were going to try to do things differently, what would that look like?*

H.   *It can sure seem that way at times. Change is harder than most of us realize. And by the way, no matter how much you change, there is always more change in store for you. The only thing in life that is predictable is change. So, literally, change will take forever in your life!*

I.   *So, right now, you are caring about not caring. Not caring is just as important a stance in life as caring, and you can choose what you care about. Let's imagine that you did care. Which way would you care?*

J.   *What feelings, thoughts, memories, and sensations are showing up for you right now? Instead of just checking out, what would happen if you just held still and let this stuff be here?*

K.   *Who am I talking to right now? The mind or the human? You don't have to accept the fact that I care about you. That is your choice. Is taking that stance right now consistent with your values? I just hope your mind is not running this show, but that you are.*

L.   *If by working, you mean eliminating all of your pain, then no, it's not working. But is feeling good the goal here, or is it to learn how feel things good?*

M.   *Given the pain you are in, I can see how you might like not to feel anything (or you might not want to feel anything). Tell me, has trying not to feel things worked to help you live a vital life?*

N.   *I know you have a number of bad feelings right now, or more correctly, you are not having these feelings right now. I keep asking because I'm trying to connect with what is showing up for you right now and to understand what you are doing with what is showing up.*

O.   *It sounds like your goals for therapy are to "feel better," not necessarily to make your life work better. Let's imagine therapy was working to make your life work better. What would you notice about your life that would tell that had happened?*

P.   *What has shown up in your life that you are not willing to make room for? It sounds like something that seems overwhelming to you. Tell me what it is that you'd rather be dead than have to experience?*

Q.   [If a suicide attempt is in progress]: *I am activating our crisis management protocol.* [After assessing that no suicide attempt is in progress]: *You know that all forms of psychotherapy are ineffective with dead people. This is an important time for you to carefully note your thoughts in your diary so we can learn from this event. I sure look forward to seeing you at our next appointment.*

4. Try to think of these statements as predictions your patient is making about what is likely to occur in the immediate future.
5. Think of ways that you could move your patient from this declaratory state of mind into a more experimental and curious state of mind.
6. Avoid overinterpreting the underlying meaning of these comments in your response. Try to stay *on the surface* and respond directly to the affect that is being presented.

Remember, do not look at the sample responses until you have completed the exercise.

The Moment of Truth: The First Crisis in Treatment

The moment of truth arrives when the issue of suicidal behavior is put directly on the table and you are in the position of either accepting or rejecting your patient's possession of the final say over whether a suicide attempt will or will not occur. The moment usually comes when increasing stress precipitates an acute suicidal crisis. This crisis can happen at any time with a repetitiously suicidal patient but is more common in the initial and intermediate stages of treatment. How you respond at this moment of truth will largely determine whether you and your patient can sustain a working relationship. You have to find a way to work together to use a problem-solving approach, often in spite of seemingly uncontrollable suicidal impulses. At this time treatment can blow apart in a showdown over whether your patient will or will not engage in some sort of self-destructive behavior.

The moment of truth is best viewed as an obvious result of the various polarizing processes that are inherent in therapy with the patient. Consequently, you are as much an antagonist as a protagonist. An acute suicidal episode is an excellent opportunity for your patient to learn how to better tolerate distressing thoughts and feelings, to see suicidality in a different context, and to experiment with new problem-solving behaviors. Some clinicians will abandon the basic treatment plan and begin to react exclusively with suicide prevention behaviors. Therapists who abandon their plan of attack in these circumstances are very likely to see their patients terminate therapy, often after a suicide attempt and hospitalization. Once consistency and predictability are lost, the likelihood of the patient's and clinician's coming back together is low.

These moments require a special devotion to duty because your patient is usually too busy *being the problem* (instead of observing the problem) to be terribly helpful. In essence, it is important to execute the treatment plan exactly as agreed to, even in the presence of the possibility of a suicide attempt. The treatment is not failing. Remember that power is limited in such circumstances. You are like a gambler holding two deuces while your patient has a royal flush. The key is not to have your hand called. When clinicians crack during the moment of truth, it is usually because of an underlying lack of conviction in the treatment. Under the threat of imminent suicidal behavior, beware of the impulse to do whatever you have to do to somehow save your patient. The more you try to assume control of the situation, the less likely your patient is to have an experience that promotes autonomy and growth. Be wary of setting up treatment plans that cannot be sustained under maximum stress. Many a clinician has been surprised by a phone call in the middle of the night concerning a patient's suicidal crisis. The answer in this situation is not an unlisted phone number or an impenetrable answering service. An emergency department physician, faced with no information from you and little knowledge of the patient, will almost always act in an overprotective (i.e., sometimes not very helpful) manner. You must be prepared for a crisis and plan for a crisis with every suicidal patient with whom you work.

A well-formulated crisis protocol about which both therapist and patient agree is essential. The protocol gives both you and your patient an agreement to fall back on and gives each of you clear responsibilities. Protocols that anticipate recurrent suicidal behavior are extremely potent because they include and make legitimate suicidal behavior a part of treatment. The protocol spells out who is to do what in the event that suicidal behavior occurs. A good protocol means you have very few *new* decisions to make when the moment arrives and can instead remain focused on executing the steps to which you and the patient have agreed.

By integrating a structured crisis protocol into treatment, your patient is able to learn experientially that you can make room for and work with suicidal behavior. With a planned, detailed, and matter-of-fact protocol in place, suicidal behavior begins to lose some of its luster, the countercontrol communication process is neutralized, and your patient is left with a clear choice:

whether or not to proceed with the behavior. As you move in a rational and controlled way into the process of responding to the patient's crisis, your patient can move in a rational and controlled way into the process of being in crisis. This approach allows your patient to cease struggling with a crisis and experience it in a more accepting way. Your patient learns to deal more rationally with things that are the inevitable consequences of being alive. One common phenomenological report from suicidal individuals is the sense of struggling to remain normal in the face of an overwhelming sense of defeat and futility. The sense of struggle ironically leads to emotional fatigue that can be tied to the emergence of suicidal impulses. When the moment arrives, you can teach your patient to drop this internal tug-of-war and work with suicidal impulses. Rather than do nothing and try to look good, your patient learns to do something constructive *and* present the appearance of working hard at it.

Resistance: An Overused Interpretation

Traditional approaches to working with the repetitiously suicidal patient emphasize that the patient's resistance has to be overcome for the patient to get better. Resistance is an enormously tempting concept, in part because it can allow you to deny responsibility for impasses in treatment. From the polarization perspective, resistance poses an interesting paradox. Whereas your therapy emphasizes learning to recognize, accept, and work with competing and contradictory beliefs your patient may have, resistance implies the patient is consciously or unconsciously using these beliefs out of a desire to stay sick. In general, clinicians use resistance interpretations when a stalemate exists. Often, one or more of the basic polarizing themes is involved. The resistance motif is often used when the patient tightens the grip on a dysfunctional belief as a counterresponse to a clinician's pushing a putatively healthier way of thinking or feeling. Resistance interpretations may also occur at the behavioral level when, for example, the patient does not complete between-session homework assignments, misses sessions, or misuses prescription medication. Some clinicians can effectively use resistance work with suicidal patients, but the danger with many resistance interpretations is that they provide a pat answer to a difficult moment and, more important, do not lead to progress. When you are tempted to sum up a troublesome impasse in therapy by attributing it to your patient's resistance, remember that if all you have is a hammer, everything tends to look like a nail. It is much more helpful to view an impasse from a variety of perspectives.

Resistance: Make It Your Problem

An alternative that can be quite helpful is to view resistance as *your* failure—an immediate and direct result of your inability to fully recognize your patient's reality. When your patient does not follow through on a particular treatment task, you may have failed to fully appreciate the limitations imposed not only by cognitive and emotional processes but also by skill deficits. For example, just asking your patient to go out and try something different, even if it is labeled as an experiment, requires your patient to have developed a particular outlook about risk taking. Why should you expect follow-through if your patient views taking risks and potentially failing as just one more predictable defeat in life? Using the language of resistance at this point not only is inaccurate but also can be a significantly destructive communication.

Is there a suffering patient in the world who would not welcome less-negative feelings? There are patients who sincerely expect failure or who believe they deserve to suffer because of past failures. This attitude is not the same as *wanting* to hurt inside; rather it addresses the fact that the patient has beliefs about getting better that may actually get in the way of succeeding. You can nonjudgmentally and objectively address a follow-through problem by *accepting blame* for failing to understand the obstacles that confronted your patient in the first place. We sincerely hope that you are in a better position to accept blame than your patient is. Once you have avoided the resistance game, a collaborative process can be developed to identify trouble spots and generate troubleshooting strategies. On another level, this technique models effective personal problem solving for your patient.

Sample Dialogue: Accepting and Working With Suicidal Communication

The following dialogue, taken from a session with a repetitiously overdosing suicidal patient, demonstrates ways of reconciling a potential transaction involving suicidal communication.

Therapist: So tell me, how has your last week been?

Patient: Well, I tried to do what you suggested. I stayed at home more and tried to find work to do that gave me more of a sense of completing things. I've been doing a lot of needlepoint work, but I still don't feel any better. I've still got all the pills I told you about, those antidepressant pills and sleeping pills they gave me at the hospital, and I know just how many to take to do what I need to do. I also know just how to take them. I won't take them all at once because I'll have trouble keeping them down, but I'll take them one by one. That way they can't pump my stomach and keep me from killing myself.

Therapist: I'm really impressed by how thorough you are in the way you prepare plans like this. How did you learn to do that?

Patient: What? What are you asking?

Therapist: I'm just impressed by how you are able to look through to the end of a plan like this. Where did you learn how to prepare a plan so thoroughly? How did you learn how to do that?

Patient: I don't know. I've always been stubborn as a mule, and I get what I want. When I think somebody is gonna try to keep me from something, I show them.

Therapist: I can tell you're a very determined person and that you know how to stick with something and see it through when you really want to get it done. By the way, have you considered how you might be dressed if you did overdose?

Patient: What the hell difference does that make? If you're dead, you're dead.

Therapist: I know, it's just that arriving at a hospital looking all disheveled would be tacky, don't you think? Also, they need to know whom to call to come and pick up your body. Have you thought about putting the name of somebody to contact in a pocket so that they would know whom to contact?

Patient: What does this have to do with my problems? You're supposed to be helping me. This isn't doing any good at all.

Therapist: I'm really sorry. Some days I'm just not as sharp as I should be, and I miss out on what is going on in a session like this. What could we do right now that would be more helpful for you?

Patient: Well, it sure doesn't help for you to be sitting here talking about me committing suicide and what I'm gonna wear and how they're gonna notify my family!

Therapist: What else could we talk about that would be more useful then?

Patient: I don't know.

Therapist: Should we talk a little while about what we could talk about that might be helpful? Does that make sense?

Patient: Well, I suppose so, but I don't think anything will help anyway.

Therapist: I know. Thinking about all the setbacks and frustrations you've had to deal with, it makes sense to expect the worst.

In this dialogue, the clinician has moved suicidal behavior off center by reconciling the push-pull contest over overdose potential. Something positive is discovered about the suicide threat, and the patient is complimented in a general way. The patient does a double take, and the clinician immediately moves to the point of resistance. The point of resistance in the dialogue is whether the patient will be allowed to "own" suicidal communications without drawing confrontation. The patient then moves to the positive point of resistance by indicating that talking about this negative content is not useful. The clinician accepts the blame for making this mistake but does not leave the point of negative resistance. The patient is asked for help in determining what would be more useful. The patient "doubles up" on the clinician by indicating that even talking about something else will not help. The clinician then moves to validate the patient's sense of hopelessness and to place it in a learning context. There is now the potential for the two of them to talk about what might work, circumventing a showdown over the patient's suicidal intent.

Providing Crisis and Social Support

The process of change for the multiproblem suicidal patient is usually slow. Slow change, however, does not mean that the patient needs weekly intensive psychotherapy. Change is a developmental process that can require episodes of therapy intermixed with linking up with competent social support. The results of the few research studies of treatment of suicide attempters suggest that longer-term supportive treatment is effective at reducing suicidal behavior per se but has little impact on underlying personality or behavioral variables. A study by Linehan et al. (1991) indicated that a 1-year treatment program consisting of weekly therapy sessions combined with group skills training was effective in reducing the number of suicide attempts and related medical costs in a sample of women with borderline personality disorder. However, few changes were noted in other basic aspects of psychological functioning. This type of programming is difficult to implement in most community mental health settings because of the high program costs being directed to relatively few patients. In addition, the durability of the treatment effects in these more intense programs is not clear. Do patients revert to repetitious suicidal behavior after the program is withdrawn? How quickly do treatment effects deteriorate? Results of an earlier study by Liberman and Eckman (1981) indicated that using a skill-oriented treatment model in a group of patients hospitalized because of parasuicide did seem to affect suicidal potential per se but did not seem to materially alter underlying personality variables such as depression, hopelessness, and problem-solving skills. Although these research efforts are not definitive, they suggest what practicing clinicians have long maintained: that the repetitiously suicidal patient needs maintenance treatment that may well span years if not decades of his or her life.

In the typical case, the initial stages of treatment consist of weekly sessions as you and your patient form a collaborative relationship and begin to reconcile polarities. Once this process has been completed, there is usually a reduction or shift in the form and intensity of suicidal behavior. At this point, you can lengthen the interval between treatment sessions (e.g., one session per month). However, your patient should always understand that more therapy can be scheduled in the event of a personal crisis as long as this move does not reinforce going into crisis. You must remain ever mindful of the potential for explosive polarizing processes. The fact that your patient is spending more and more time out of therapy is not an indication per se that effective problem solving has been learned and suicidality is no longer an issue.

Effective Management: A Therapeutic, In-System Perspective

A major part of the formula for success with the repetitiously suicidal patient is to develop an effective approach to ongoing self-destructive behavior. To accomplish this task, you must effectively manage how adjunctive and ancillary services are delivered to your patient. In working with the chronically suicidal patient you often wear many hats: clinician, case manager, advocate, and care coordinator. The more you plan these roles, the less likely there is to be confusion and a critical change of course during a crisis.

The Therapeutic Management of Chronic Crisis

A well-known feature of repetitiously suicidal patients is the capacity to slip in and out of crisis: the *crisis-of-the-week syndrome*. With some regularity, you are presented with a crisis by the patient that invites diversion from the treatment plan. These crises often occur in association with suicidal or self-destructive behavior. To some extent, these crises are the hallmark of the early phase of treatment. You need to assimilate these events into the flow of therapy without losing continuity or placing yourself and your patient in a confrontational or adversarial position.

Many of the important components of a behaviorally based crisis management protocol are discussed in Chapter 7 ("Managing Suicidal Emergencies"). The repetitious suicide attempter requires special attention to and stringent application of these principles. The reason is simple. You are going to be confronted with more suicidal behavior, and you need to have a very potent yet flexible plan of attack. The issue of the patient's engaging in suicidal behavior or experiencing severe crisis needs to be addressed at the outset of treatment. You need to be able to predict these events. You need to make very clear your particular stance with respect to intervening in suicidal behavior. The ground rules about after-hours phone contact and scheduling extra sessions in relation to suicidal behavior must be clear and mutually acceptable. You must work together to develop a crisis card so your patient can begin learning to activate natural social supports. Encourage your patient to make therapeutic contacts *before* engaging in any self-destructive behavior. Create a structure in which you and your patient can effectively deal with the chaos and distress that often go along with suicidal behavior. The structure allows you both to hark back to earlier agreements as a guide to managing your way through these difficult times.

A well-prepared crisis protocol will answer nearly all the questions in advance. The existence of the protocol creates a higher level of comfort in the midst of suicidal behavior and generally promotes healthy interventions. The patient who is scared but locked-in on suicidal behavior is drawn to a calm and purposeful clinician. An effective crisis plan can provide an experiential demonstration that selecting alternatives to uncontrolled self-destructive behavior can be rewarding. *Assimilation of crisis* is a major case management strategy. Many events that trigger suicidal crises in the chronically suicidal patient are small in scale and are better thought of as the straw that broke the camel's back. If the suicidal response is taken off center stage, the patient may discover straightforward and effective ways of solving the specific event. When the suicidal behavior *itself* becomes the focus of attention, then it is

very difficult to solve primary problems—the problems that have pushed suicidality to the forefront.

Beware of Magical Assumptions

The clinician often communicates overtly or covertly an expectation that the
patient's suicidal and self-destructive behavior will either disappear or rapidly
diminish as a simple consequence of entering treatment. In this scenario, it is
assumed that the "magic" of therapy will immediately effect a change in the
patient's suicidal behavior independent of the therapeutic approach. Consequently, a recurrence of suicidal behavior is viewed as a signal that treatment
is failing. Negative therapeutic processes can result from this error (e.g., resistance interpretations, anger and confrontation, and ultimatums). The major
philosophical cornerstone of effective case management is to use the suicidal
crisis as an opportunity to promote growth in the patient. It is easy for the
clinician's patience to wear thin when the covert expectation of decreased suicidal behavior is continually being violated. The act of planning and frequently reaffirming the crisis management plan in collaboration with the
patient will help neutralize this potentially destructive dynamic.

Case Management in the Community

Case management activity is an essential ingredient of effective treatment of
chronically suicidal patients. It is important to conduct case management at
key points of contact, particularly with emergency department providers,
who may not have the necessary clinical skills to independently implement an
effectual treatment response to a repetitiously suicidal patient. Because suicidal behavior is potentially life threatening and raises legal liability issues, it
is imperative that your case management plan be as specific and concrete as
possible. For example, most emergency departments have rotating shifts of
personnel, which means that the repetitious suicide attempter may not see the
same medical provider despite repeated contacts. The case management plan
needs to transfer easily from one shift to another. Thus it must be written in
the patient's chart in concise and concrete language. The plan should identify
who the patient is, the nature of the patient's suicidal behavior, a rationale for
the management plan, and the specific steps providers are to take in the event
that they come into contact with the patient after a suicide attempt.

Figure 6–1 presents a sample emergency department case management plan for a repetitious drug overdose patient. The goal of the management plan is to limit psychotherapeutic interaction with the patient after an index suicide attempt, in that such interaction is a powerful reinforcement of suicidal behavior. Conversely, more attention, caring, and support are made available if the patient presents to the emergency department before engaging in the self-destructive behavior. The most difficult part of forming such plans is to get health care providers to understand the rationale for, and importance of, stabilizing and then discharging a repetitious attempter after an index episode. This idea is both new and scary to most health and mental health professionals, who often believe this approach flies in the face of risk management rules. The tendency is to hold the patient until mental health personnel eliminate all suicidal ideation or secure a no-suicide contract and then to discharge the patient. This method results in a tremendous amount of interpersonal attention, which can promote a positive view of suicidal behavior in your patient.

Case management plans frequently require repeated contacts with both medical and mental health personnel at key contact sites. The need for repeated contact is especially prominent when the patient tests the case management plan by increasing suicidal behavior and presentations for care. Providers become uncertain and worried about legal liability. In such cases, it is important to teach providers about the learning theory concepts of extinction and spontaneous recovery. *Extinction* means that when suicidal behavior is neither positively nor negatively reinforced, it will gradually decrease in frequency. However, well-learned behaviors undergoing extinction can spontaneously reappear at an even higher frequency for short periods. Suicide attempting may initially increase but will gradually decrease as the extinction plan is consistently followed.

When *spontaneous recovery* occurs with a suicidal patient, medical or mental health personnel often are caught off guard. Spontaneous recovery is a critical point in determining the overall integrity of the case management plan. The more participating providers know what to expect in terms of the suicidal patient, the easier it is to draw attention to the fact that predicted events are occurring. This approach provides the reassurance needed for providers to drop their own biases about how to treat suicidal patients and can allay risk management concerns.

TO: MSWs, RNs, MDs, Consulting RNs, Medical Clinics, Emergency Centers

RE: Protocol for S.L.

As most of you know, S.L. has made multiple medication overdoses. None of these attempts have been lethal, few have been serious. We are trying to modify her behavior without reinforcing it and without teaching her to be more lethal. We request that when she presents to you with an overdose, you respond in the following manner:

1. Assess medical danger.
2. Treat her medically, as necessary.
3. Provide S.L. with a meal, but otherwise limit interaction to the bare minimum. Provide no positive or negative feedback. No punishments, no lectures. Your contact with S.L. should be a noninteractive event.
4. Send S.L. home after treatment and a meal.
5. All therapeutic interactions are to be with N.S., S.L.'s primary therapist only.

For further concerns or questions, please contact N.S. If N.S. is not available, contact O.S., the clinical backup in this case.

Thank you for your help with this difficult client.

Figure 6–1.   Management protocol for S.L., a repetitious drug overdose patient.

Someone Has to Be in Charge

A final critical feature of effective case management is identification of a single provider who makes the final decision about the patient's care. This individual also handles all psychotherapeutic transactions with the patient. This individual ordinarily is the patient's primary therapist. The goal of all such funneling actions is to restrain providers at other contact points from delivering uncoordinated treatment—often treatment that is incompatible with the approach being followed by the primary therapist. This aspect of treatment is especially critical when a behavioral model is being followed and when reinforcements of the suicidal behavior are the all-important issue. In return for keeping interventions within set boundaries, the primary therapist needs to respond promptly to requests for help by participants in the case management plan. If the primary therapist is going on vacation, other members of the case management network need to be aware of the absence so they do not expect help that cannot be delivered. Case management plans often fall apart during a therapist's absence, insofar as the patient may interpret the therapist's departure as a form of abandonment and go into crisis.

When the various treatment entities properly funnel decisions to the primary clinician, the clinician is able to extend a wider umbrella of protection for the patient if the patient complies with the behavioral treatment plan. In other words, you can control the reinforcements offered at a wider variety of contact points (i.e., hospital emergency departments, primary care clinics, and community mental health center emergency teams). When the system works, the patient does not have two sets of response rules applied with regard to suicidal potential. This plan allows the clinician and patient to work with a consistent crisis management model.

To Hospitalize or Not to Hospitalize?

Many suicide attempters admitted to an inpatient psychiatric facility have a history of at least one previous suicide attempt. As "dangerousness to self" increasingly becomes a reason for hospitalization, inpatient staff may feel that they are dealing with a revolving door filled with repetitious suicide attempters. These admissions raise the question of how hospitalization should or can support the treatment process for the repetitious patient. Of all the subpopulations of suicidal patients, this one is probably the most difficult to deal with effectively during an inpatient admission. The patient is often not well liked by hospital staff and tends to be at disproportionate risk of a discharge against medical advice. The patient may be given the diagnosis of borderline personality disorder before the first intake interview, because repetitious suicidal behavior itself is strongly related to such a diagnosis. In the era of managed health care, few inpatient units can offer the long-term treatment programs that even begin to address the many cognitive and emotional needs of a multiproblem patient with borderline personality disorder.

An equally important consideration is that the repetitiously suicidal patient is often dumped into the inpatient system by a frustrated clinician who just wants the patient to go away. When we talk about a therapist "cracking" in the moment of truth, this type of dumping is one of the cardinal manifestations. The clinician is tired of the patient and hands over care to an inpatient staff that then may be negatively disposed toward the patient because of the dump and the out-of-control gestalt that develops around poor planning. Consequently, the suicidal patient can evoke a high level of hostility and confrontation during even a brief hospital stay. This patient may well receive less preferred and less intensive forms of treatment available on the unit. The patient may be given a medication regimen that has little chance of succeeding. Diagnostic and treatment disputes often erupt between treatment team members (i.e., "splitting") and are blamed on the patient rather than on the real culprits: interpersonal conflicts, disciplinary jealousies, and turf struggles among members of the treatment team.

Even when none of the negative consequences occurs, consider also the possible reinforcing effects of the hospitalization per se on the individual's suicidal problem-solving potential. The patient is removed from a stressful environment and is exposed to a highly structured setting in which all basic needs are met. Positive caring and attention are forthcoming from the unit staff. The individual feels looked after and supported because of the suicidality, and, accordingly, the behavior is reinforced. In all, hospitalization potentially offers negative and positive reinforcement scenarios. Given the frequent use of hospitalization for suicidal persons, this reinforcement may be a factor in the relatively high risk of suicidal behavior in the United States.

There are certainly circumstances in which a patient is bound and determined to land in some type of intensive care facility. The clinician cannot ignore this possibility in effective treatment planning. It is therefore critical to attempt to develop alternatives to traditional inpatient treatment in the event the patient ends up in that part of the treatment system. This plan may involve contracting with a local hospital to allow the patient to elect a 72-hour voluntary time-out with an automatic prearranged discharge plan. If the local community has an acute care crisis facility, the patient can be directed to seek admission to that facility with prearranged, short-term problem-solving goals. Your goal is to eliminate the reinforcement potential from any intensified treatment and, as soon as possible, get the patient back into the natural environment and in the right mind-set to solve problems.

Continuity in case management is particularly critical during the transition between inpatient and outpatient mental health treatment. When a suicidal outpatient enters a psychiatric hospital in the context of a suicide attempt, there is an even greater need to coordinate in a way that supports the basic outpatient treatment plan. The reason is simple: Psychiatric units can deliver an enormous array of services in a very condensed time. If these services are not synchronized with the outpatient treatment regimen, long-term treatment can suffer. Psychiatric inpatient staffs have their own way of dealing with suicidal patients and often do not coordinate with the outpatient system. Coordination usually occurs at the initiative of the primary therapist. Because the very act of admission to a hospital is a potent reinforcement of suicidal behavior, the primary therapist must make efforts to arrange for appropriate treatment at likely inpatient sites.

It is important to provide a sound rationale to attending psychiatrists to gain support for a treatment plan that may be different from the usual milieu plan of the unit. For example, if the plan calls for automatic discharge within 48–72 hours and a minimum of psychotherapeutic contact, the responsible physicians need to understand why that is the best way to care for the patient. The primary therapist needs to initiate the dialogue about how best to coordinate the interface between outpatient and inpatient care. There are myriad reasons why this type of coordination and planning may not happen, and it is sometimes particularly difficult to effectively work together with the repetitiously suicidal patient. To deal with coordination of care, try to establish a consistency of purpose with at least one inpatient psychiatric site, and direct the patient to that site in the event of a suicidal crisis. Discourage admissions to hospitals where the staff seems unwilling or unable to coordinate care. Hospitalizations are helpful when they reinforce your long-term strategy, but they are harmful when they subvert it. In Chapter 8 ("Hospitals and Suicidal Behavior") we discuss additional aspects of hospitalization and provide inpatient treatment techniques.

Helpful Hints

- The repetitiously suicidal patient differs in degree, not kind, from episodic and more functional patients.

- The mechanisms of repetitious suicidal behavior are the dominance of ineffective rule-governed responses, emotional avoidance, lack of behavioral flexibility, and specific skill deficits.
- The goals of treatment of the repetitiously suicidal patient are the same as those in treatment of the acutely suicidal patient: teach acceptance and tolerance of emotional pain and problem-solving skills.
- Building patterns of committed, valued action that are the antithesis of the suicidal lifestyle is the ultimate goal of treatment.
- With the repetitious patient, the therapist must reconcile polarities that develop over who is in control.
- Effective treatment avoids confrontations with the patient over a variety of issues related to ongoing suicidal behavior.
- The repetitiously suicidal patient typically needs ongoing intermittent crisis and supportive care because beliefs and behavior are very slow to change.
- In case management, it is important to establish an open, direct dialogue with the patient about how suicidal behavior will be responded to in the course of therapy.
- Intersystem case management is a basic therapeutic function and requires collaboration with emergency departments, crisis units, and inpatient psychiatric units.
- In general, inpatient hospitalization is not helpful for the repetitious patient; consider using short-stay, acute care alternatives.

References

Kreitman N: Parasuicide. New York, Wiley, 1977

Liberman RP, Eckman T: Behavior therapy vs insight-oriented therapy for repeated suicide attempters. Arch Gen Psychiatry 38:1126–1130, 1981

Linehan MM, Armstrong HE, Suarez A, et al: Cognitive-behavioral treatment of chronically parasuicidal borderline patients. Arch Gen Psychiatry 48:1060–1064, 1991

Strosahl K, Chiles JA, Linehan M: Prediction of suicide intent in hospitalized parasuicides: reasons for living, hopelessness, and depression. Compr Psychiatry 33:366–373, 1992

Selected Readings

Beck A, Freeman A: Cognitive Therapy of Personality Disorders. New York, Guilford, 1990

Evans J, Williams JMG, O'Loughlin S, et al: Autobiographical memory and problem solving strategies of parasuicide patients. Psychol Med 22:399–405, 1992

Farmer RDT: The differences between those who repeat and those who do not, in The Suicide Syndrome. Edited by Farmer R, Hirsch S. Cambridge, UK, Cambridge University Press, 1979, pp 192–204

Hawton K, Catalan J: Attempted Suicide: A Practical Guide to Its Nature and Management. Oxford, UK, Oxford University Press, 1982

Hayes S: Comprehensive distancing, paradox and the treatment of emotional avoidance, in Paradoxical Procedures in Psychotherapy. Edited by Ascher M. New York, Guilford, 1989, pp 184–218

Hayes S, Jacobson N, Follette V, et al: Acceptance and Change: Content and Context in Psychotherapy. Reno, NV, Context Press, 1994

Hayes S, Strosahl S, Wilson K: Acceptance and Commitment Therapy: An Experiential Approach to Behavior Change. New York, Guilford, 1999

Hayes S, Barnes-Holmes D, Roche B: Relational Frame Theory: A Post-Skinnerian Account of Language and Cognition. New York, Plenum, 2001

Jones B, Startup M, Jones RSP, et al: Dissociation and over-general autobiographical memory in borderline personality disorder. Psychol Med 29:1397–1404, 1999

Linehan M: Cognitive Behavioral Treatment of Borderline Personality Disorder. New York, Guilford, 1993

MacLeod AK, Williams JMG, Rose G: Components of hopelessness about the future in parasuicide. Cognit Ther Res 17:441–455, 1993

Sidley GL, Whitaker K, Calam RM, et al: The relationship between problem solving and autobiographical memory in parasuicide patients. Behav Cognit Psychother 25:195–202, 1997

Startup M, Heard H, Swales M, et al: Autobiographical memory and parasuicide in borderline personality disorder. Br J Clin Psychol 40:113–120, 2001

Strosahl K: Cognitive and behavioral treatment of the personality disordered patient, in Psychotherapy in Managed Health Care: The Optional Use of Time and Resources. Edited by Berman W, Austad C. Washington, DC, American Psychological Association, 1991, pp 185–201

7

Managing Suicidal Emergencies

More on Crisis and Case Management

In this chapter we provide you with the tools you need to manage a suicidal crisis in a way that is collaborative and leads to good results. We will show you how to coordinate care across different parts of the same delivery system and across different service delivery systems. We include this separate chapter on crisis and case management because this aspect of your work with suicidal patients is the most demanding. The patients not only are higher-functioning, acutely suicidal patients whose cases you must appropriately assess and manage over the short run but also are suicidal patients prone to slip in and out of crisis over the course of treatment. Dealing with episodically or chronically elevated suicidal behavior makes most providers ill at ease. In contrast to the traditional notion of crisis intervention with all of its risk management implications, *crisis management* refers to the act of planning, in collaboration with your patient, a response to either the immediate suicidal episode or the possibility of recurring suicidal behavior. The goal of planning is to establish a framework that rewards alternatives to suicidal behavior and minimizes short-term reinforcements both in the

175

present situation and if suicidal behavior recurs.

The complexity of effective crisis management is due to the same factors that make suicidal behavior a multidimensional entity. Some patients you encounter will be in the midst of a highly contained suicidal crisis that is clearly the result of life stresses (e.g., divorce, discovery of a terminal illness, death of a spouse, or being fired from a job) or a discrete episode of a treatable mental disorder. The patient's premorbid level of functioning is high, and substantial social support may be available. At the other end of the crisis management continuum are patients who are always experiencing some degree of suicidal thoughts or behaviors, although the intensity level will usually vary from week to week. Although they follow the principle that one cannot downplay the significance of any suicidal communications or behavior, these two kinds of presenting situations require different clinical responses. For example, it is not productive to view repetitive and intractable ideation as a suicidal crisis per se. For a substantial number of suicidal patients, suicide ideation is a daily reality—it is an ever-present symptom. These patients are often assigned to case management systems. The case manager and therapist must continually balance their crisis intervention response to the recurring suicidal behavior, ongoing treatment, and the community resource needs of the patient. On the other hand, the patient with no appreciable history of suicidal ideation and no attempts would be regarded as being in suicidal crisis. The notion of crisis means a significant upturn in suicidality to levels well beyond the previous typical range of that behavior in that individual. So, yes, a chronically suicidal patient can exhibit a suicidal crisis, but the crisis must entail levels of suicidal ideation or behavior that are significantly increased above the levels typically manifested by the patient.

We Are All Case Managers

Case management is best defined as the effective coordination of care through a variety of settings. A case manager addresses liability issues, overcomes system-level obstructions, communicates a clear treatment plan, and deals with resistance other providers may experience in following through with case management strategies. A significant goal of case management, and sometimes the most difficult goal to reach, is to resolve the potential conflict of interest between the social control goals of immediate family members or the treatment system and your own sense of what is in the patient's best interest. Anyone involved in the treatment of a suicidal patient will find some aspect of case management embedded in his or her work.

Remember, whereas crisis intervention is largely a matter of interaction between you and your patient, case management is your attempt to influence the behavior of others to support your patient. These two missions often converge with patients who are less responsive to treatment. Repetitious suicidal patients typically need more episodes of behavioral management as well as more frequent and active case management. When case management demands intensify, you must be aware of a tendency to drift away from a problem-solving focus. In effective treatment, problem solving and emotional tolerance must be pursued consistently, regardless of recurrent crises or the amount of case management.

Working Through Suicidal Crises: Five Principles

Whenever a patient needs help with a suicidal crisis, successful intervention relies on the following five principles:

1. Suicidal behavior is designed to solve specific problems that your patient views as inescapable, interminable, and emotionally intolerable. Any of us can become suicidal when faced with these conditions. Successful crisis intervention helps the patient work through the suicidal crisis by using both short- and intermediate-term problem-solving strategies.
2. Your demeanor plays a critical role in accelerating or decelerating the crisis. Approach the suicidal crisis in a direct, matter-of-fact, and candid manner and avoid appearing nervous, scared, or apprehensive about what may happen next.
3. Nearly all occurrences of suicidal behavior are nonfatal. Most suicidal crises do not lead to suicide. Furthermore, there is little evidence that any form of crisis intervention, be it counseling, psychopharmacology, or both, will prevent suicide. Most of the therapeutic maneuvers that count are based on the assumption that the patient will be alive tomorrow. The patient should learn from this crisis and by this experience be less vulnerable to subsequent crises. If your only motive is to keep the patient alive, a precious opportunity for human growth will be missed. With the recurrently suicidal pa-

tient, you will do little but react to a never-ending stream of suicidal episodes unless your patient is able to grow and learn from each episode.

4. Real suicidal crises are self-limiting. Few individuals can maintain an acute crisis for more than 24–48 hours without going into an adaptive period of emotional exhaustion. Your treatment should be focused on getting through the next 1 or 2 days while anticipating that the episode will soon give way to the underlying problems that provoked the crisis.

5. The final objective in crisis intervention is to help the patient solve problems in nonsuicidal ways. Your intervention techniques should never reinforce suicidal behavior. Your goal is neither to punish nor to reinforce suicidal behavior but to make it a "neutral valence" event. By achieving this valence, the suicidality will lose any advantage it has over other more adaptive problem-solving strategies.

Working Through Escalating Suicidal Behavior: Strategies

There are specific strategies to use when working with an acutely suicidal person. These techniques can be put into play with both new patients and individuals in ongoing therapy. They are outlined in Table 7–1.

The most important thing to remember is that you need to remain calm, direct, and methodical. Your demeanor helps promote the gathering of certain important pieces of information, such as your patient's perception of the problems that have precipitated suicidal behavior, the range of problem-solving responses that have been considered, and mood and cognitive factors that will influence short-term problem solving.

Part of your assessment of your patient's problem-solving flexibility is to monitor for the presence of psychotic or thought-disordered symptoms. In general, the more disordered a patient's thinking, the less workable is a self-directed problem-solving plan. A psychotic illness always must be treated. A patient with a psychotic illness may benefit from the increased structure of short-term hospitalization or from longer-term hospitalization that targets the underlying psychotic symptoms.

Assessment of mood-related symptoms is an important step in understanding the patient's crisis. Mood-related symptoms strongly influence a patient's motivation and energy level. A severely depressed patient is likely to have trouble following through with a problem-solving plan because the energy is not there to accomplish it. A highly anxious, agitated patient has plenty of energy to expend but may experience trouble focusing on a plan of attack. Mood is the highway to a reading of your patient's suffering and desperation. The reading will help decide whether the initial plan is aimed at teaching the patient to tolerate suffering or is focused on solving the problem or problems that triggered the crisis.

It is important to assess your patient's current use or potential for abuse of alcohol and drugs. Many suicidal people use alcohol or drugs as a way to deal with emotional pain. If drug or alcohol abuse plays a role, avoid lecturing or moralizing about the negative effects of substance abuse. Instead, form a problem-solving plan that is incompatible with the passive approach that leads to drug or alcohol use, abuse, or dependency. For example, schedule constructive activities during the time your patient is prone to drink or take drugs, or consider follow-up calls at a time when your patient might be tempted to use. Ask about high-risk times when drugs or alcohol were not used. Find out how your patient was able to devise better solutions, and then focus on the increased use of these strategies. It is often useful to enlist the aid of others in your patient's social network to help restrict access to alcohol and drugs and to support or initiate activities that are incompatible with heavy use. If a drug or alcohol program is available, encourage and assist your patient in enrolling.

Do not assess your patient's potential for suicidal behavior by limiting yourself to the use of traditional suicide risk assessment questions. These traditional risk factors have not been shown to be accurate predictors of the risk of suicidal behavior. There are much more revealing ways to assess the likelihood that your patient will remain suicidal. These questions are relatively simple to ask and are included in Table 4–1 (Key factors in assigning risk for suicidal behavior). You should probe the patient's outlook in the following areas:

- The patient's belief in whether suicidal behavior would solve problems
- The patient's ability to stand or tolerate significant emotional pain
- The patient's reasons for not committing suicide should the opportunity present itself
- The patient's ability to see a future that is positive and life enhancing
- The patient's history of using suicidal behavior as a means of solving problems

Table 7–1.   What to do when the crisis heats up

A.   Be direct in questioning about suicidal behavior.

B.   Be calm and methodical—remember functional analysis.

C.   Review mental status. Ask about psychotic symptoms, mood symptoms, and drug and alcohol abuse.

D.   Schedule extra contacts if necessary, but beware of reinforcing suicidal behavior—emphasize problem solving, not "feeling better."

E.   Try to help the individual generate short-term objectives.

F.   Now is a great time to make a "random" support call.

G.   Negotiate a positive action plan.

H.   Review the crisis protocol.

Reframe suicidal behavior in the problem-solving context so that your patient's first impression of treatment is oriented toward solving real-life problems. This approach helps remove the stigma of suicidal behavior and gets your patient thinking about symptoms from a different perspective. Work hard to get the message across that suicidal behavior is not a sign of abnormality but that suicidal behavior is an outcome of a legitimate problem-solving process. This tactic in itself will help defuse a suicidal crisis.

The Positive Behavior Action Plan

The desired outcome of effective behavioral management is a short-term plan that has been *collaboratively* generated by you and your patient. The plan addresses what actions need to be taken in the succeeding days to solve the problems that precipitated suicidal behavior. A good plan is easy to define. *It is concrete, detailed, and within the patient's ability.*

The two most common mistakes in this endeavor are, first, forming a plan that the patient is unable to accomplish, and second, pushing a plan that is not formed by a collaborative effort. Given the pressure inherent in the crisis situation, you understandably want the outcome to be good. Beware of your tendency to define *good* solely by what you think the patient ought to be doing to solve difficulties. Your kind of good may not be something that your patient agrees with or is able to do. It is not necessary to make major changes to solve problems. Achieving a *small positive step* can have as great an impact as trying to make a heroic change in life. Remember, the psychology of suicidal behaviors is that the situation is viewed as unchangeable and inescapable. Any positive change can bring these rigid assumptions into question. When you and your patient have developed a workable short-term plan, you have done your best to ensure that your patient will succeed. Tailoring a plan to a patient's capability is the key ingredient of success. If the plan is unachievable, your patient will give up and have one more failure with which to deal. The plan must be seen as workable and, if successful, as a positive step forward. Two key questions are

1. "If you were able to do X in the next few days, would you see that as a sign of progress?"
2. "Do you think X is something that you can actually do in the next few days, given the way you are feeling?"

The following are some typical goals for the short-term problem-solving plan:

1. Look for ways to decrease your patient's social isolation.
2. Increase pleasant or reinforcing events.
3. Engage, or engage again, your patient with an activity in which success is likely.
4. Increase the patient's physical activity level through some type of exercise.
5. Increase the patient's use of relaxation strategies or self-care behaviors.
6. Get the patient to engage in coping responses that have worked in previous times of crisis.

An isolated person may have a competent social support network but worries about being a burden and so avoids interaction. In this situation, a short-term behavioral plan might emphasize initiating a social contact with one or more helpful persons but limiting the amount of time spent talking about personal problems. You can work on ways to get your patient to resume a pleasant activity that has somehow dropped out of the weekly routine. The method may be scheduling one or two walks in the park over a 5-day period, going to a movie, or taking an aerobics class. It is often useful to look for coping strategies the patient has used in previous times of travail. Was it taking a nice warm bath each night? Practicing meditation or simple relaxation strategies two or three times a day? Calling a friend in another city for a daily check-in? From a strengths-based perspective, you want to look for what the patient already knows how to do. It is easier to reinitiate existing behaviors than it is to learn new behaviors. The scale of these interventions is not large, and the interventions themselves may not directly target suicidal ideation or behavior. The important point is to choose interventions that are likely to be done. Initially, actually experiencing some success is much more important than struggling to solve huge problems. Whenever possible, this short-term, constructive plan should be written down, and follow-up contact should be scheduled so you and your patient can assess how the plan is working. This follow-up session is usually conducted 1–3 days after the initial intervention. Many providers find that this follow-up contact can be a simple phone call at a prearranged time, just to assure that the plan is being followed and no un-anticipated barriers have surfaced. Of course, the patient understands when leaving the initial meeting that he or she can return immediately for care if the plan backfires.

The No-Suicide Pact: Who Is the Beneficiary?

Over many years, the no-suicide pact has made its way into clinical lore as a way to remove the threat of suicide. Patients are asked to state in writing that they will not engage in suicidal behavior for a set period. The no-suicide pact was originally conceived as an inpatient management technique. It has subsequently been used in other settings and situations, often, unfortunately, with scant effort directed at evaluating efficacy or even examining theoretical underpinnings. Some systems unfortunately have used this pact as a hospitalization plan (i.e., to be discharged, one has to promise not to be suicidal). Other systems use a patient's refusal to sign as a criterion for involuntary hospitalization. The no-suicide pact can deceive the clinician into believing that the patient's condition has improved. No research studies have shown that suicide is less likely in people who have agreed to a no-suicide pact or that this strategy reduces suicidal behavior over the long term. Theoretically, this contracting could increase risk of suicidal behavior if the patient is not able to abide by the agreement, feels guilty, and does not disclose this fact to the therapist.

The no-suicide pact has been used as a requirement for transfer from one treatment system into another system. Would you require a depressed person not to be depressed in order to be discharged from an inpatient setting? If the depressed person were able to be nondepressed simply because of that type of pressure, would the patient not have been relieved of depression already? If the suicidal patient were really able to agree not to be suicidal, would it not seem reasonable to assume that the patient would already have made such an agreement? Patient flow between parts of a comprehensive system of care needs to be based on assessment of the level of intensity and need, not on extraction of a statement that can have a misleading and soporific effect on clinicians.

The alternative to the no-suicide pact is the positive action plan. In brief, patients are asked to engage in positive, constructive behaviors for a defined interval. This change in emphasis, from what you should not do to what you should do, can become a critical part of an effective problem-solving set. Remember, *no* strategy guarantees the removal of suicidal potential. Your goal is to create a positive context for short-term problem solving.

The Emotional Tone of the Intervention

Although the stated goal of crisis intervention is to develop a problem-solving set and formulate a plan, it is important to remember that the underpinnings of suicidal behavior are emotional desperation and intolerable and inescapable pain. You need to validate these difficulties and provide effective support. Crisis intervention sessions can go bad when the therapist's anxiety to do something leads to disconfirmation of the patient's sense of pain and distress. The "just do it" motif might work well in the locker room, but it is anathema to a suicidal patient, who may interpret this attitude as an overwhelming injunction. Reacting to such an injunction, your patient may well become more suicidal. When this reaction occurs, your patient is saying to you, "No, you don't quite understand just how badly I'm really feeling. Let me show you a little more directly!" As frequently as you can, validate your patient's sense of emotional pain and your understanding that the patient is considering suicide as an option to stop the pain. At the same time, state with confidence your belief that if the two of you work together, better solutions can be found. There are many technical steps that can be taken with a patient who is suicidal, but the emotional tone of the session is by far the most important mediator of overall success. The patient who feels listened to and accepted is more likely to carry through with a collaborative problem-solving plan.

Managing Suicidal Behavior During Treatment

Any patient may become suicidal again during the course of therapy, given the right set of life events or a predisposition to use suicidal behavior as a problem-solving device. Although this possibility seems obvious, some clinicians seem to implicitly assume that the act of entering therapy causes suicidal behavior to disappear. If suicidal behavior reappears, the danger is that a clinician with this mind-set is often unprepared and angry and will confront the patient. The art of successful therapy is to collaboratively anticipate and plan for the recurrence of suicidal ideation or behavior at some point during treatment. The act of coming for treatment is not to be confused with solving real-life problems. Acknowledge this fact. This acknowledgment will put your clinician-patient relationship on a realistic level rather than perpetuating an idealized image of therapy. Use any recurrence of suicidal behavior as a learning laboratory for problem-solving skills and emotional pain tolerance. This technique gives the patient permission to bring everything into the treatment session rather than withholding information that the patient believes will displease the clinician.

Suicidal Behavior Protocols

Table 7–2 lists important points to cover when developing a behavior-based protocol for managing suicidal behavior. Most of the protocol is established in the initial part of treatment. The following three things are important:

1. The protocol is well understood and agreed to by your patient.
2. The protocol is consistent with both your and your patient's beliefs and values.
3. The patient views the protocol as a fair and workable arrangement.

The bottom line is the answer to the question, What are you, the clinician, going to do if I, the patient, become acutely suicidal? Your patient may, for example, be concerned that you will use involuntary hospitalization, may be fearful of that, and so may be reluctant to mention anything about a suicidal crisis. Accordingly, you must state your beliefs and values regarding a potential suicidal crisis. Legal, ethical, and moral crosscurrents in this situation

Table 7–2.   Protocol for managing suicidality during therapy

A.   Prevent alcohol and drug use.

B.   Reward appropriateness.

   1.   Do not reinforce suicidal behavior with increased attention.

   2.   Reward attempts to address crisis without suicidal behavior.

C.   Establish a specific crisis protocol for each patient—the crisis card strategy.

D.   Remember that suicidal thinking and behavior continue after hours—consider crisis clinic, social support network.

E.   Establish conditions under which the individual may seek hospitalization.

   1.   Emphasize self-control behaviors over acting-out behaviors.

F.   Make clear your own policies regarding involuntary hospitalization.

can influence the success or failure of therapy. This information should be discussed openly. Any joint action plan must reflect principles that you are willing to follow in the midst of a suicidal crisis.

Using Hospitalization

Your strategies for using hospitalization should be laid out. This plan might include discussing the issue of short-term acute care, voluntary admissions for evaluating diagnostic issues, and the use of involuntary admissions. For example, you may present the value of voluntary, short-term, time-out admissions over longer-term, vaguely defined admissions. The goal is to build a scenario in which effective decision making can occur in the event of a crisis by including your patient in the planning and thereby maximizing the sense of his or her self-control.

Scheduling Additional Sessions

Additional sessions may be needed in the event of a suicidal crisis. However, scheduling additional sessions may inadvertently reinforce suicidal behavior by making your extra attention seem a reward for being suicidal. This problem is an ongoing one with many of the usually unscheduled interventions that occur during periods of elevated suicidal behavior. In general, it is more helpful to schedule additional sessions when positive problem-solving behaviors are occurring and your patient will benefit from more intense work. If additional contacts are required because of a crisis, try to make the contact as minimally intensive as possible. Use techniques such as brief follow-up phone calls rather than 1-hour, face-to-face visits. Focus efforts on reinforcing and building constructive problem-solving behaviors. Encourage your patient to develop self-sufficiency in crisis—the internal ability to weather the storm.

Receiving Telephone Calls

Establish very early in treatment when and under what conditions you will receive unscheduled calls. Once the patient has *initiated* suicidal behavior, limit your participation in crisis phone calls. A good strategy is to indicate that in the event suicidal behavior has already occurred, you will undertake an assessment of medical lethality. If you believe the patient is in medical danger, an emergency aid car will be sent to the location immediately. Indicate that this is not an appropriate time to discuss more effective problem-solving options, and reinforce your interest in discussing the situation at the next regularly scheduled session. Encourage your patient to make mental or written notes concerning the handling of this particular crisis, and strongly state your belief that there is much to be learned from this situation. If your patient calls regarding thinking about a suicide attempt, always offer the opportunity to dispose of the means, and engage in a brief problem-solving discussion. Again, instruct your patient to make notes and bring them to the next session, and praise your patient about calling you instead of pursuing suicidal behavior. Never be abrupt or imply that you are punishing your patient because of misbehavior. Many practitioners cringe at the thought of cutting short a phone call, fearing the liability implications if the patient ever committed suicide. This dilemma is the result of liability-based treatment. The issue is to look at what *works clinically* in this situation; document the basis of your decision and the steps you have taken to help the patient.

In general, crisp handling of phone calls coupled with turning the context of the phone call into a homework assignment is far more constructive than lengthy unstructured conversations.

A problem in taking phone calls is that you, like anyone else, need rest, time away from work, and the ability to pursue other activities. You want your patient to call you before initiating suicidal behavior. This approach builds self-control and personal responsibility. When your patient complies with this protocol, you should be available to consult at any hour of the day. It is important, however, to remind your patient that clinicians, like all people, have nighttime and after-hours activities that are not a part of their daytime work.

Agree on the rules beforehand, and let your patient know how you will respond in various situations. If your activities are under way when a patient calls, indicate that you are busy, instruct the patient to follow the self-support plan on his or her crisis card (see later, The Two-Part Crisis Card), and schedule a time to talk that will work for both of you.

A more perplexing situation is when your patient calls, is suicidal, has the means immediately present, and tells you, "I'm going to do it!" In this case, instruct the patient to remove the means from immediate access by turning it over to a friend or otherwise disposing of it. At times like this, it is helpful to say something like, "I want to help you, but it is going to be hard for us to talk if you are thinking about killing yourself at the same time. Let's put that stuff aside so we can work together to sort out what is going on here." If your patient will not agree to your request, then any phone-based problem solving is likely to be a melodrama, and a bad one at that. You have already indicated what your stance is in situations like this. Now is the time to follow through, and now is the time to respond to the crisis card.

Making Random Support Calls

Inform your patient that from time to time you will be calling to see how things are going. The random support call strategy is designed to remove the association between escalating suicidal behavior and your attention. The random support call neutralizes this association and can be a precipitant for major movement in therapy. The random support call is usually very short, no more than 2–3 minutes. The essence of the message is, "I care about how you're doing. I hope the behavioral homework assignment is going well. You were going to pay particular attention to X. How is that going? I really look forward to seeing you next week. Take care." In other words, do not perform therapy on the phone, but rather support your patient in whatever activities are occurring that week. To make this process truly random, you might want to randomly draw numbers and then set up a schedule 3 months in advance. These calls will be made regardless of your patient's functional status. Random support calls do not have to be made often; one a month can often have a positive impact. When your patient is in a crisis, you can bend the rules a bit and add an additional call or two to reinforce the problem-solving strategies that your patient is currently using. Even though your patient is in a crisis, the message is essentially the same, and the duration of the call is short (2–3 minutes). This strategy creates a new kind of relationship. The issue of mattering to someone and being understood can be so central to your suicidal patient's view of the world that a simple 2-minute call may be a major event in treatment.

The Two-Part Crisis Card

The last and most important crisis protocol strategy is developing a crisis card.

Identification of Resources

The first part of the crisis card is identification of resources. The goal is to teach your patient to use existing social support and community resources and to depend less on you as time goes on. Identify one or more competent and supporting persons who can be contacted in the event of a crisis. A competent social supporter is a person who will not lecture, cajole, or moralize about problems but will provide emotional validation and a safe atmosphere. Once these social supporters are identified, your patient writes down their names and phone numbers on a card.

Some patients will have trouble identifying a social support group. They may not know many people. They may hold back from this task because they feel they are already too much of a burden to others in their life. At these times consider meeting with your patient and family members or friends who might provide effective support, and develop a structure to which all can agree. For example, if long, rambling, and somewhat painful conversations have been the rule, suggest a time limit (e.g., 5 minutes) and a couple of points to be covered in that time frame. The self-support strategies on the crisis card (see later, Second: Self-Support Strategies) can always be incorporated in the points to be covered. Encourage all parties to be creative and come up with a support solution that is helpful and comfortable for everyone.

Next, identify community resources who can be contacted in the event of a crisis. Examples include the local crisis clinic, a mental health center emergency services unit, and a local emergency department social worker. These resources are written down along with their corresponding phone numbers. The last name on the card is yours, with associated work and home numbers. Your patient is to contact all of the listed social supports first and then contact the community resources. If those resources fail, your patient is to contact you. The two of you agree that you will be as available as possible for such contacts if the patient has followed through with attempts to contact all of the other resources. If your patient has not followed the protocol, then (directly and in a supportive way) ask the patient to proceed through the card and call back if all attempts at contact fail to ameliorate the crisis. If your patient is unable to follow this procedure, proceed as described earlier (see Suicidal Behavior Protocols), but emphasize the need to reexamine the protocol at the next session.

Development of Self-Support Strategies

The second part of the crisis card is development of self-support strategies. Two to four instructions can be quite helpful. If substance abuse is an aggravating problem, the card item could be, "Don't drink. If I am drinking, stop drinking." Simple tactics for affect regulation are useful, such as, "Take 10 deep breaths and count to 50." Positive statements, to be repeated several times, can be useful, such as, "I am a strong person and have weathered moments like this before." Last, and perhaps always, evoke the problem-solving perspective, for example, "I need to step back and look at the problem I am having right now." An example of this type of crisis card can be found in Chapter 10 ("Suicidal Patients in General Health Care"), Figure 10–1.

Growing Through Suicidal Behavior

Two key principles can make any occurrence of suicidal behavior a productive event. *First, suicidal behavior in the midst of therapy is not evidence that the treatment is failing.* It simply means that the behaviors that brought the patient into therapy in the first place are still present in the patient's problem-solving repertoire. The clinician who insists that the patient refrain from suicidal behavior in order to continue therapy is doing a disservice. You must learn to harness your disappointment regarding a patient's suicidal crisis. A good place to start may be to remember that although your ability to influence is great, your power to control is quite limited.

Second, the basic goal is to neutralize the reinforcement of suicidal behavior. When your patient presents you with suicidal behavior, you have a golden opportunity to directly modify the behavior. In other words, you arrange consequences so your patient will not experience suicidal behavior as a potent problem-solving strategy. For example, if a patient uses the hospital to escape his or her environment (i.e., I am suicidal, let me in), then develop other forms of respite. If suicidal ideation or behavior helps to relieve anxiety, then devise strategies for installing alternative methods of achieving anxiety reduction. If your patient is dependent on you and uses suicidal behavior to maintain an unhealthy intensity of treatment, then adhere to a regular session schedule and do not reinforce suicidality with additional contacts. If anything, look for periods of good, nonsuicidal problem solving to schedule additional contacts.

The neutralizing interventions depend on your assessment of how suicidal behavior is being reinforced. What does your patient get out of being suicidal that allows the behavior to continue even with its longer-term negative consequences? Remember, despite the social stigma attached to suicidal behavior, it is a very powerful short-term problem-solving strategy with strong internal and external consequences.

Be consistent with the acceptance- and value-based problem-solving model. A clinician who abandons a treatment model during suicidal crises has a much greater likelihood of failure, either through unsuccessful therapy or through premature termination of treatment. The key is to show the patient that everything comes down to accepting what is there to be felt while engaging in effective problem solving whether a crisis is present or not. The more matter-of-fact, candid, and upbeat you are when confronting recurrent suicidal behavior, the more likely it is that your patient will adopt this mental set and become task oriented instead of focusing on avoiding emotional pain. Use the assessment strategies described earlier (see Working Through Escalating Suicidal Behavior: Strategies). Build homework assignments on tracking suicidal ideation or behavior. Identify trigger situations. If your patient can experientially verify these concepts, then his or her view of suicidal behavior will change.

Your patient can become demoralized over the recurrence of suicidal behavior, believing it demonstrates that things have not changed for the better. The more direct, matter-of-fact, and accepting you are of the suicidal behavior, the less likely it is that your patient will take any of these negative interpretations to an extreme. Many a patient has dropped out of therapy in an effort to avoid the disappointment of, or a confrontation with, the therapist.

You must know the difference between working with suicidal behavior in a constructive way and inadvertently reinforcing it. Learn the difference by focusing on problem-solving communication and pain tolerance as twin frameworks for therapeutic transactions. Pay less attention to suicidal behavior per se, except as it relates to experiments in problem solving. This process can be difficult because of the power of suicidal communication. It can be difficult to remain as interested in problem-solving communication as it is in suicidal communication. Do you sit perched on the edge of the seat when the patient is talking about suicide but relax and sit back when problem solving is the focus of exchange? Be alert to your nonverbal intensity and whether anything increases your focus when the discussion moves away from suicidality. To combat this phenomenon, assess the amount of time spent talking about acceptance, willingness, and effective problem solving versus suicidal behavior. The general rule is that at least 85% of the session should be spent in the former pursuit and no more than 15% spent focusing directly on suicidal behavior.

When suicidal behavior recurs, you need to execute the agreements formed in the initial sessions. This step is a test of your belief in the treatment protocol because the protocol is being challenged under real-life conditions. This point is where "the rubber hits the road," especially with the chronically suicidal patient. If you have a soft spot, it will be revealed now. If you have promised the patient that no involuntary hospitalization will be used but now invoke this intervention, you have jeopardized the working relationship. When soft spots appear, modify the treatment plan to be consistent with what you really believe. You must be genuine. Admit your mistakes and ambivalence, renegotiate the plan, and push on.

To Hospitalize or Not to Hospitalize: That Is the Question

No examination of crisis intervention or case management principles would be complete without addressing the issue of voluntary or involuntary psychiatric hospitalization as a treatment of suicidal crisis. Hospitalization is overused for suicidality. In Chapter 8 ("Hospitals and Suicidal Behavior") we address the plethora of factors that must be understood to use this modality appropriately. These factors dictate a cautious approach to the use of hospitalization as a behavior management tool. The emphasis should be on whether psychiatric hospitalization is the preferred treatment of an underlying mental illness that is related to the patient's suicidal potential. For example, a schizophrenic patient who is experiencing command hallucinations to commit suicide would profit from a secure environment so that medications could be started with the expectation that the command hallucinations would begin to dissipate with effective treatment. The focus is not suicidal behavior per se but the underlying mental disorder. When a person is hospitalized to treat the illness and suicidal behavior is present, it is important to closely monitor reinforcement patterns on the unit so that suicidality is not being exacerbated.

Emphasizing Responsibility and Self-Control

Patients who take responsibility for hospitalizing themselves before engaging in suicidal behavior are usually demonstrating at least a mild form of appropriate value-based problem solving. The experience can enhance the sense of self-control, and this type of admission is often viewed favorably by inpatient staff, thus setting the stage for a positive therapeutic encounter. For these reasons, it is important to work to place responsibility for the admission in the hands of your patient, so that the admission is an act of self-control and thus a positive problem-solving event. Your patient can be instructed that it is a positive act of self-control to acknowledge that a time-out is needed. In the event a patient wants a time-out hospitalization, the patient should go (not be taken) to the appropriate emergency or intake unit and request a short-term stay with an anticipated discharge in 48–72 hours. The goal is to minimize time away from the environment in which the real problems are occurring while allowing the patient to form a problem-solving plan. This approach encourages use of personal responsibility and self-control to offset the potentially negative effects of a hospitalization.

There are too many situations in which clinicians tend to treat their anxiety about a patient's suicide risk rather than securing appropriate treatment of the patient. Inpatient staff members sometimes feel that suicidal patients have been "system dumps" because clinicians up the line simply are too anxious to deal directly with the problem. The result is that anger is directed at the patient for being the one who caused the mess in the first place. The charge to outpatient clinicians is to seek appropriate consultation to reduce their anxiety about a particular patient and then to gear treatment strategies to the best interest of that patient. Therapy is not a vehicle for reducing clinician anxiety. The goal of therapy is to help patients solve problems using clinically effective strategies.

Case Management: Crisis Intervention at the System Level

When a patient receives medical or mental health treatment from different systems or is seeing more than one provider within a single system, case management concerns almost inevitably arise. For example, a suicidal patient may first visit a family practice physician's office and then be transferred to an emergency department for an assessment. At this point, the patient is either hospitalized or referred to the outpatient mental health system for counseling. Each of these contact points represents both an opportunity for coordinated care and a potential for conflicting, disjointed, and idiosyncratic responses. Effective case management is an attempt to ensure that treatment is consistent as the patient crosses between systems or moves between levels of care within a system while keeping each service delivery entity working within its own area of expertise. In other words, each player knows his or her role and what he or she is supposed to do and not do.

When systems work closely together, case managers play a crucial role in coordinated transfer planning. Local delivery systems need to be part of a coordinated and interconnected network that will provide various services to the suicidal patient. Case management is responsible for coordinating the patient's smooth transition between systems. The inpatient psychiatric facility shares responsibility for the patient's continuous and coordinated care in the outpatient system. Outpatient treatments are likewise coordinated through the inpatient stays in a way that ensures consistency in the care models being used with the patient. When it transfers a patient into inpatient or outpatient care, the emergency department should effectively encourage the patient to follow through with the referral. The emergency department should coordinate its delivery of services with any outpatient or inpatient unit that has previously worked with the patient. This model may bedevil risk managers who want to protect their agencies but are not aware of the principles of quality clinical care. However, in this model the community of systems is the treating agent, and a highly efficient managed care format results.

There are many instances in which drawing an arbitrary line between systems or departments and providing no effective communication between these entities invites negligence. Had the facility in question seen itself as part of the treatment community, that extra phone call might have been made to ensure that the patient had followed through with an appointment at another facility. The potential negligence was not the patient's state of mind on leaving the facility. The negligence was that the facility did not do its best to get the patient to the next destination. When the patient makes a coordinated transfer between and within systems, quality of clinical care increases exponentially. Providers in different systems can talk with one another without feeling put on the spot or exposed to unacceptable risks. Not only does the patient benefit, but also fewer resources are expended in the process. Better outcomes, lower costs, and less litigation sound like a good equation.

The Concept of Funneling: Someone Has to Be in Charge

Most effective case management systems have a single person who is accepted as being in charge of coordinating treatment and transfers. This person may be the therapist or the crisis interventionist or the mental health professional who is attempting to move the patient to various needed treatment locations. Our clinical experience suggests that a treatment plan is likely to fail when it does not identify a single professional in charge of care management decisions. Funneling is the act of building case management protocols that return the patient to a single provider. Other providers who have contact with the patient are asked to follow the care management instructions developed by the provider in charge. Done appropriately, funneling prevents splitting (disputes between members of the treatment team), inconsistent or contradictory responses to suicidal behavior, and confusion on the part of the patient.

Although the funneling type of case management can be time consuming, it is a legitimate and indispensable component of effective treatment. You must talk with other health and mental health practitioners so that they understand the rationale of treatment and are willing to follow the role that is scripted for them. This approach is particularly true with suicidal patients because everyone not only has strong reactions to suicidal behavior but also may have a variety of ideas on how to work with the patient. The result can be an array of conflicting treatment approaches that leave the patient bewildered and confused. Similarly, the pressure to fix the patient can lead to dissension among providers who conflict with one another about the right way to treat suicidal behavior.

In many treatment settings, case management is not viewed as part of legitimate clinical service delivery. Time spent in case management activities may be counted as administrative time by a clinic manager. This attitude puts the clinician in the position of being negatively reinforced for implementing perhaps the most important aspect of treatment. In effect, the time spent comes out of the clinician's hide; caseload expectations remain the same despite the difficulties associated with managing a particularly suicidal patient. This organizational stance not only invites negligence claims but also reduces general quality of care.

Qualities of the Effective Case Manager

Three pivotal interventions define an effective case manager with the suicidal patient.

1. You need a clear approach to the problem, and you need to articulate this approach and explain to others in the treatment system how it will produce clinical benefit.
2. You need to state in concrete operational terms what various players must do to support a coordinated treatment effort.
3. You need to provide frequent feedback about how the plan is working, and you need to deal with the concerns of the various providers.

The dearth of literature on how to treat suicidal patients causes many therapists to have vague case management goals. This vagueness results in confusion among other providers or among clinical team members who understand neither the objectives of the treatment nor what they are supposed to do to support those goals. In the worst-case scenario, this lack of clarity does not surface until suicidal behavior escalates and the patient begins traveling within or across systems. When this movement occurs, providers initiate their own strategies and are unwilling to abandon their strategies in favor of ones they do not completely understand or endorse. Effective case management requires that you be absolutely clear about the treatment strategies that will produce a good clinical outcome. Clarity is provided with a written case management plan that is distributed to all concerned parties. Figure 7–1 is a model case management planning sheet that helps begin to address an effective case management plan.

Armed with a therapeutic strategy, the therapist still needs to convert that strategy into concrete instructions for different health and mental health care providers. These instructions need to be consistent with the skills and background training of the providers. For example, instructions for emergency department physicians might focus more on issues related to medical evaluation and short-term instructions about transferring care of the patient if further assistance is needed. Expecting emergency department physicians to perform social work services or psychotherapy with a suicidal patient is usually not realistic.

It is important for you to provide a constant flow of feedback, both positive and negative, to key points in the system. Ironically, most case management discussions occur when things are not working. The tension associated with these discussions can be ameliorated if there is balance between positive and negative feedback. Take the time to call back providers who followed instructions and show them how their contribution has helped produce a good clinical outcome. If a provider's efforts supported continuity and coordination of care, the provider should be made aware of that fact. In other words, try to avoid circumstances in which the only communications with other providers occur when there are disagreements about treatment strategies or a failure to follow through on a specific plan.

A good example is developing a strategy to make suicidal behavior a neutral valence behavior. This behavior requires the providers who contact the suicidal patient to respond neither with excessive attention, caring, and concern nor with punishment, confrontation, and cajoling. This task is difficult in the heat of the moment. When there is good adherence to this approach in the emergency department, it is very important to let providers know they did a good job.

An equally important goal of effective case management is to have the patient understand that the case management umbrella will be user-friendly as long as the patient stays underneath it. Many patients with character disorders or other oppositional attributes test the timbre of a case management system. The patient presents with suicidal ideation or behavior at various points in the case management system to see if there is consistency in the response.

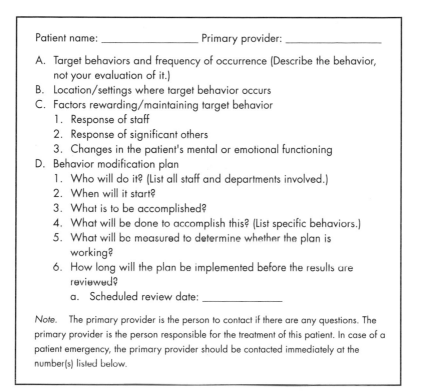

Patient name: _____ Primary provider: _____

A. Target behaviors and frequency of occurrence (Describe the behavior, not your evaluation of it.)
B. Location/settings where target behavior occurs
C. Factors rewarding/maintaining target behavior
   1. Response of staff
   2. Response of significant others
   3. Changes in the patient's mental or emotional functioning
D. Behavior modification plan
   1. Who will do it? (List all staff and departments involved.)
   2. When will it start?
   3. What is to be accomplished?
   4. What will be done to accomplish this? (List specific behaviors.)
   5. What will be measured to determine whether the plan is working?
   6. How long will the plan be implemented before the results are reviewed?
      a. Scheduled review date: _____

Note. The primary provider is the person to contact if there are any questions. The primary provider is the person responsible for the treatment of this patient. In case of a patient emergency, the primary provider should be contacted immediately at the number(s) listed below.

Figure 7–1. Sample suicidal behavior management protocol.

If the patient has collaboratively developed the case management plan with the therapist, there will be less testing. However, it is important to have the patient understand the limits of the case management system. For example, it is difficult to link every emergency department and hospital to a particular patient's case management plan. The patient needs to understand that presentation at an uninvolved facility could result in an unpredictable outcome, such as involuntary hospitalization or the use of restraint and seclusion. The patient must understand that the therapist cannot control what will happen outside the umbrella. The goal is to get the suicidal patient to go to service delivery sites where the practitioners have been prepared to respond in a clinically effective manner.

As it is with providers, it is important to praise the patient for staying within the case management umbrella. The therapist may bend over backward to be available for a crisis call in such a circumstance. This extra attention will reinforce the patient for sticking with the case management plan. Although it may be an inconvenience, this aspect of management generally takes a lot less time than managing a care plan that is being continually tested by the patient.

Suicidal patients differ in the extent to which they need case management services. Difficult patients need much more case management than do other patients. Difficult patients tend to be more disordered, multiproblem patients who may have developed a lifestyle of chronic suicidal crisis. If you are willing to follow the principles outlined in this section, there is a greater likelihood that service delivery systems will respond in a way that not only helps the patient but also makes life easier for the therapist.

Helpful Hints

During Crisis

- The two key skills in effective crisis intervention are validating emotional pain and forming an effective problem-solving plan with the patient.
- One goal of effective crisis intervention is not to prevent suicide but to help the patient learn how to move through problems and tolerate negative affect.
- Another goal in crisis intervention is to stay consistent with the problem-solving model while focusing on short-term goals.
- Try to defocus on a suicidal behavior per se while increasing emphasis on solving specific problems that precipitated the crisis.
- Remember that almost all true suicidal crises are short-lived, no longer than 48–72 hours.
- Beware of using psychiatric inpatient treatment for suicidal behavior per se because it may inadvertently reinforce the behavior.

In Therapy

- In therapy, directly address and plan for the possible recurrence of suicidal behavior during the initial session with the patient.
- Develop a well-rounded case management plan that involves providers with whom the patient may have contact over time.
- When planning for crisis, emphasize steps that reinforce the patient's responsibility and self-control in seeking help.
- Analyze reinforcements for suicidal behavior so that interventions do not inadvertently reinforce suicidal problem solving.
- Effective case management with other service delivery systems requires a clear statement of treatment goals, concrete instructions for other providers, and frequent provision of feedback.
- The most effective case management plans identify a single provider who is in charge of the patient's care and related clinical decision making.

Selected Readings

Bancroft J, Skirimshire A, Casson J, et al: People who deliberately poison themselves: their problems and their contacts with helping agencies. Psychol Med 7:289–303, 1977

Blumenthal SJ: Suicide: a guide to risk factors, assessment, and treatment of suicidal patients. Med Clin North Am 72:937–971, 1988

Bongar B, Berman A, Maris R, et al (eds): Risk Management With Suicidal Patients New York, Guilford, 1998

Chiles J, Strosahl K: The suicidal patient: assessment, crisis management and treatment, in Current Psychiatric Therapy. Edited by Dunner D. Toronto, ON, Canada, WB Saunders, 1993, pp 494–498

Chiles JA, Strosahl K, Cowden L, et al: The 24 hours before hospitalization: factors related to suicide attempting. Suicide Life Threat Behav 16:335–342, 1986

Kleespies P, Deleppo J, Gallagher P, et al: Managing suicidal emergencies: recommendations for the practitioner. Prof Psychol 30:454–463, 1999

Newscom-Smith J, Hirsch S (eds): The Suicide Syndrome. London, UK, Croom Helm, 1979

8

Hospitals and Suicidal Behavior

A Complex Relationship

Hospitalization is overused as a treatment of suicidal patients. When hospitalization is used, it is often for the wrong reasons. American psychiatric practice, and the legal structure around it, has given the hospital a pivotal role in dealing with a suicidal person, and yet as a treatment for suicidal behavior, hospitalization has limited usefulness. As the era of health care reform and managed care continues in the United States, the role of the psychiatric hospital in mental health has changed. Gone are the days when a patient could be hospitalized for weeks or months while the hospital took responsibility for offering the primary treatment a suicidal individual was going to receive. Most hospital stays now are held to a week or less. Faced with this changing practice and the financial crisis it has precipitated, many psychiatric hospitals have either closed or converted psychiatric beds into medical-surgical beds. More important, this restriction in the use of psychiatric services requires that inpatient units reevaluate their role in relation to the outpatient delivery system. In our view, the hospital plays an important role but one that is secondary to the delivery of outpatient mental health care. More than ever, it is imperative that hospital staff communicate with outpatient providers and engage in patient care strategies that are consistent with existing outpatient treatment plans.

As painful as this transition has been for the inpatient sector, it may be a change for the better as far as the treatment of the suicidal patient is concerned. There is little evidence that a stay on a psychiatric unit has a long-term beneficial effect on suicidal behavior. No reasonably well-controlled studies have demonstrated that hospitalization will reduce suicide potential. Furthermore, there is little or no agreement about a set of criteria that should be used for hospitalization. In some settings most suicidal patients referred to emergency departments are not psychiatrically hospitalized, whereas in other settings most suicidal patients are hospitalized. More and more, hospitalization in response to suicidality is driven by legal concerns, concerns that are predicated on a rather vague notion of what one must do to avoid malpractice litigation. This approach is unfortunate, because hospitalization is an extremely important component of a multitiered psychiatric crisis response system, and the crises include suicidal crises. Hospitalization is one of several essential tools to have in your treatment toolbox. Hospitalization can become problematic when it is viewed as the *only* response you, the clinician, can make to a suicidal patient. An old adage is pertinent: if all you have is a hammer, you must treat everything as if it were a nail. In this chapter, we examine first the negative and then the positive aspects of hospitalization. We describe treatment principles and discuss alternatives to inpatient treatment.

In the United States, all states have a mental health statute that requires a clinician to initiate hospitalization or other strong protective measures if a patient is deemed at *imminent risk of suicide.* Although there is a wide range of personal opinion about a person's right to commit suicide, this opinion is not expressed in most state statutes. There is no doubt that the social control function of the law is strongly in favor of stopping the individual from committing suicide. Furthermore, the assumption behind most state statutes is that hospitalization, whether voluntary or involuntary, represents the most effective short-term preventive treatment of suicide. Individuals who are deemed imminently suicidal are thus deprived of their civil right to be free of detainment and coercive treatment so that short-term intervention in their suicidal crisis can be provided. Several questions are raised by involuntary treatment. First, does placement in a psychiatric unit prevent a person from engaging in or succeeding at suicidal behavior? Second, does hospitalization represent an effective treatment per se for a person who is suicidal at the time of admission? Third, are there long-term consequences associated with being psychiatrically hospitalized that can be potentially detrimental to a suicidal person (i.e., can hospitalization make things worse)?

Does Hospitalization Prevent Suicide?

There is little conclusive evidence to suggest that being placed on a psychiatric unit reduces a person's chance of committing suicide in either the short or the long term. Suicides occur more often on psychiatric units and in jails than in any other location. Inpatient suicides account for as many as 5% of all known suicides. Adding this figure to events in the first week following hospital discharge accounts for as many as 11% of all suicides. Both jails and psychiatric inpatient units contain troubled individuals who may well consider the setting and its restraints an intense invasion of their personal freedom. This sense of invasion may increase emotional distress, be perceived as yet another problem, and create or add to the pressure to use suicide as a solution. That the suicide rates in psychiatric units are not the *lowest* in the land suggests that individuals who are intent on the act are able to complete it even in the midst of staff concern and close observation.

Almost all mental health care workers have heard anecdotal reports of inpatient suicides. Mental health professionals with some expertise in this area frequently receive legal requests to be expert witnesses in situations in which patients on psychiatric units have succeeded in killing themselves. Many of these anecdotes and descriptions are reminiscent of scenes from movies such as *Stalag 17* and *The Great Escape,* in which the central theme of the film is the incredible cunning and resourcefulness of individuals who are determined to escape observation and do what they feel they have to do. Although most psychiatric hospitals have fairly elaborate protocols for close observation of at-risk patients, the inability to accurately predict risk level means that many closely observed patients are not those who commit suicide. Almost all mental health workers with inpatient experience know of patients categorized as being at low or declining risk who have gone on to attempt or complete suicide.

Does Hospitalization Work?

The second question has to do with the efficacy of hospitalization in dealing with suicidal ideation or suicide attempt. No outcome studies have shown that the inpatient location per se is a critical factor. Researchers who have looked at the treatment of suicidal patients in the inpatient setting tend to confound the setting with the type of treatment actually delivered. Often these treatments could have been delivered just as well in an outpatient environment. Results from inpatient clinical outcome reports are at best equivocal and at worst do not support this level of intervention. Germane to the potentially negative impact of hospitalization are a variety of research findings that show suicidal patients tend to be received in a less than favorable way by hospital staff. The patient receives less-preferred forms and amounts of treatment and may have interactions hallmarked by confrontation and hostility. These negative reactions may help explain the elopement or discharge against medical advice undertaken by as many as 50% of hospitalized suicidal individuals. A problem in reviewing articles on efficacy is the lack of clear clinical characteristics of suicidal persons who are hospitalized versus those who are not hospitalized. Probably crucial to the successful use of a hospital is a judicious process for selecting admissions.

When hospitalization occurs because no other options are available, a variety of bad reactions can set in. The patient can feel abandoned. The staff can feel angry because it appears that outpatient clinicians are not doing an adequate job. Both patient and staff can feel frustrated and disconnected from what went on before and what should go on after. These reactions can produce their own ill effects and muddle the meaning of outcome information.

Iatrogenesis: The Unintended Side Effects

Hospitalization has unintended side effects. As a rule, the most invasive treatments have the most invasive side effects, and hospitalization is no exception.

First, labeling can determine behavior. People live up or down to the labels that are attached to them. The label *psychiatric patient* can lead to a negative view of self that is confirmed in subsequent behavior. The experience of being in an inpatient facility is something the patient may never forget, even when the stay is positive.

Second, admission highlights the issue of autonomy. When the essence of a suicidal crisis is a struggle with one's sense of self-control over suicidal impulses, then the decision to hospitalize can be a potent communication that the patient is out of control, thus confirming his or her worst fears. It important to present hospitalization as a component of a rational multimodal treatment plan, not as a last-ditch effort because all else has failed. Never give the message that if hospitalization does not produce change, there is nothing more to offer.

Third, hospitalization can act as reinforcement for suicidal behavior. This result is the most troubling unintended effect of hospitalization. We believe it explains the pervasiveness of repetitive suicidal behavior among patients hospitalized for suicidal behavior. By providing short-term relief from long-term problems, hospitalization can reinforce the patient's sense that suicidality works (i.e., "I made a suicide attempt and things got better"). Hospitalization removes the individual from a stressful situation, and the subsequent anxiety reduction can reinforce the recurrence of suicidal ideation or behavior. The patient moves from an environment marked by hostility, criticism, or confrontation into, we hope, an environment of caring and concern. In a hospital with a good therapeutic milieu, much of the conflict the patient has been experiencing is carefully governed in the hope that this strategy will protect the patient's psychological stability. Troubled relationships seem to improve. For example, someone admitted for a suicide attempt is suddenly reconciled (at least temporarily) with a formerly hostile, alienated spouse who may feel blame for the way things have gone. After an adolescent's suicide attempt, a dysfunctional family can be galvanized around the patient's suicidal behavior in a way that seems as if the family is coming together. Because most of the possible negative consequences in these scenarios are longer term (e.g., other people avoid you, spouses get even more angry) and therefore not readily apparent, the patient may feel empowered to solve problems using suicidal behavior again.

Most inpatient units are struggling with the growing number of repetitious suicide attempts. In one study (Chiles et al. 1989), we found that the mean number of previous suicide attempts among persons hospitalized for suicide attempts was more than two. As the number of attempts increases, staff members may begin to feel pessimistic about their interventions. This attitude can lead to a dispirited sense of resignation among staff members that can produce conflict and hostility in staff-patient relationships.

Architecture: Is This Place a Hospital or a Prison?

In addition to the psychological and interactional elements, the architecture of the unit can be a major factor in determining inpatient efficacy. Some hospital wards, particularly older ones, are designed to maximize isolation rather than to promote observation. Can nurses be aware of activities from a central station? Is staff at ease about a patient's location and behaviors so that therapeutic work can be done? Without a spacious, commodious, and eminently viewable unit, there is danger that ward staff will overuse suicidal precautions as a means of patient control. Wards full of nooks, crannies, and blind spots (and many of them are) create a nearly guard-prisoner relationship between staff and patient. This atmosphere does not promote, and in fact demotes, the goals of successful treatment of suicidality: autonomy, efficacy, and self-control. Keep these components in mind. If you have a choice of inpatient services, visit them. When you are involved in hospitalization, try to admit your patient to the unit that is the most efficiently unobtrusive. If you are fortunate enough to have a say in new unit construction or old unit remodeling, insist that clinical criteria be incorporated into design.

Will I Get Sued if I Do Not Hospitalize?

There continues to be much clinical lore about the role of hospitalization as a way to prevent lawsuits. Our experience as expert witnesses over nearly two decades suggests hospitalization does not prevent lawsuits. A good plaintiff's attorney intent on prosecuting a lawsuit will find something that you did "wrong," so do not carry around any illusions that because your patient is hospitalized you are somehow off the hook of legal culpability. More important, *you cannot predict which patient will commit suicide, and there are not enough beds to hospitalize everyone troubled by suicidal behavior.* Almost every clinician working in an area of mental illness treatment has close knowledge of suicide occurring during treatment. For a therapist directly involved, the death of a patient can have a devastating effect. What could I have done differently? can become a painful and obsessive question for the clinician, just as it can be for friends and family. The accusation, "You should have hospitalized," can feed into troublesome second-guessing. The fear that a lawsuit will begin when a patient dies haunts many health care providers. Of course, a dispassionate reading of the literature can equally support an accusation of, Why did you hospitalize? followed by a powerful self-doubt, "I should not have hospitalized." Can you be sued for inappropriately hospitalizing? It does not happen often—not yet—but fear of such lawsuits could become another worry.

Performing legally sanctioned interventions may not be the same as performing good treatment. There can be a discrepancy between what is stated in the law (a legislatively conceived attempt at health care) and what seems the best and most appropriate clinical way to approach the problem. Decisions made *primarily* to address liability issues are often not good treatment decisions. In the litigious climate of the United States, lawsuits can happen at any time and for any reason. The question is not, Will I get sued? The question is, Have I used my training, experience, knowledge, and expertise to devise a treatment plan that can help my patient deal with the problem of suicidality? Think clearly, and document your thinking. *If you do not write it down, it did not happen.* Have a reasonable treatment plan and stick with it. Make sure that your clinic and hospital document risk management criteria that you believe represent sound practice and then follow those criteria. *Never* be in the position of having to state that you did not know what those criteria were.

When Hospitalization Goes Sour

The case report literature is full of examples of individuals who are hospitalized because of suicidality. This literature contains little or no long-term follow-up statements about the benefits of hospitalization. The following is a case report of an individual whose suicidal behavior escalates after hospitalization.

> Ms. T, a 28-year-old white woman, worked in a laboratory in a major medical center. Soon after beginning employment, and 2 years before her first hospitalization, she sought treatment for depression and relationship difficulties. At that time she spoke of her parents' strictness and told of a difficult childhood. She was born and raised in a small town, the oldest of six children. Her parents were active members of a fundamentalist church. The family was often in financial difficulty, and Ms. T was working and giving her paycheck to her parents by the age of 13. Both parents demanded that she take over a number of child-rearing duties, and they frequently blamed her for troubles

with her younger siblings. The parents would often go to religious retreats, leaving Ms. T in charge. Ms. T had little time or inclination for a social life and worked throughout her high school and college years. When she reached adulthood, Ms. T's parents continued to demand that she support the family, including buying clothing for her siblings. At one point Ms. T took over payments for her father's truck. Just before she entered treatment, Ms. T's parents had gone on a prolonged trip. When they returned, they found that some of their other children had gotten into difficulty. They called Ms. T, who was living in another city, and blamed her for her failure to "come home and look after her brothers and sisters."

Ms. T was treated with antidepressant medication, and supportive psychotherapy was conducted at a rate of approximately one session every 2 weeks. Ms. T's first visit to an emergency department came when her physician was on vacation. Ms. T complained of increased depression, anxiety, and suicidal thoughts. She was living alone but had supportive friends, several of whom had urged her to go to the emergency department. Ms. T had tried but could not get hold of the individual covering for her vacationing caregiver. The emergency department physician evaluated her as being in "imminent danger of suicide" and strongly recommended hospitalization.

Ms. T did not do well in her first 4 days of inpatient treatment. She became quite distressed over the needs of the other patients. The psychiatric symptoms did not improve. When asked, Ms. T stated she still "felt" suicidal. The antidepressant medication was continued, and benzodiazepines were added to the regimen. On day 5 of hospitalization, Ms. T demanded to leave, stating she needed to return to work. At that point, she was involuntarily committed at a state hospital. She was there for approximately 1 week and then discharged to her outpatient provider. The psychotherapy was continued in the original format: supportive sessions every 1–2 weeks. In approximately 1 month, Ms. T called her psychotherapist at night stating that she had cut her wrists. An ambulance was dispatched, and Ms. T was again admitted to a local hospital. She argued about staying and was transferred involuntarily to the state hospital. Ms. T was discharged after approximately 3 weeks. Ten days later, she once again contacted her psychotherapist stating she had made a suicide attempt. This time she had taken approximately 1,500 mg of a tricyclic antidepressant and had severely slashed her right arm. The medical treatment required several days of inpatient cardiac monitoring. The self-inflicted wound required 28 stitches.

We do not know what would have happened to Ms. T if that first emergency department visit had gone differently. Would an alternative plan have provided adequate health maintenance until her primary physician returned?

We do not know, and hindsight often is not fair. However, in this case, hospitalization of the suicidal person did not decrease the behavior and in fact may have had dramatic negative consequences. Did Ms. T have a devastating loss of self-control? Did social stigma and loss of civil rights have a profound effect on her identity? Were suicidal precautions and one-to-one close observations invasive and counterproductive? Was the sense of intense scrutiny that comes from ubiquitous staff presence experienced as oppressive, and did that scrutiny induce restlessness and frustration? For Ms. T, did any of these negative emotions and behaviors outweigh any benefit that suicide precaution might have had in providing a temporary aura of safety? Was Ms. T received less favorably by staff?

Staff-patient interactions can be confrontational and abrasive with mutual hostility, anger, and mistrust. This intense environment can affect the judgment of both staff and patient. For many staff members, it is difficult to analyze provocative behavior and at the same time try to rapidly respond to it. One staff member can act in a way that other staff members might disagree with, and staff-staff conflict can ensue. Considering these factors, there are times the hospital atmosphere does not engender good therapeutics.

When Should You Hospitalize a Patient?

Although hospitals are an important part of the clinician's armamentarium, a decision for hospitalization should be carefully weighed. Remember that there is no evidence that hospitalization reduces long-term suicide risk or that hospitalization is an effective treatment for suicidal behavior per se. In cultures in which hospitalization for a suicide attempt is less of an option, there may be less overall repetitious suicidal behavior. Psychiatrists need to be aware that few medication regimens have been proved to reduce suicide risk. At the time of this writing, only clozapine has been shown to lower the rate of suicidal behavior and only in patients with schizophrenia. Medications should target psychiatric syndromes that are known to respond to those medications. With these caveats in mind, we recommend three criteria that can be used to decide about hospitalization: *the presence of a serious psychiatric illness, the need for short-term sanctuary, and the use of hospitalization to reshape suicidal behavior.*

Psychiatric Illness

The most easily justified reason for admission to a hospital is the presence of a serious psychiatric illness that requires the intense therapeutic and evaluation milieu of a hospital setting. Schizophrenia, severe affective disorders, and psychotic depressive disorder are just a few of the psychiatric conditions that could benefit from the around-the-clock management that only hospitals can provide. Another advantage of hospitals is the concentration of diagnostic facilities that can be rapidly brought to bear. This array of services can be crucial in understanding a severely disturbed or distraught person who might be experiencing one of a number of illnesses or toxic states. Finally, more than one thing can be wrong. It is increasingly common to find individuals who have two or more conditions contributing to their distress. Most common is the combination of a psychiatric illness and substance abuse disorder. Inpatient services can put several treatments into action at the same time and can do so at a time of crisis and urgency when a person might be most amenable to change. This ability to implement treatment quickly is a notably good component of units that are able to take this dual (or more) diagnostic and holistic approach. Although treating an underlying mental disorder or substance use disorder is a legitimate reason for admission, remember that treating those conditions is not the same as treating the patient's suicidal risk. Many hospital programs are so overly focused on managing suicidal risk that the delivery of effective treatment of underlying conditions is compromised.

Short-Term Sanctuary

A second reason for hospitalization involves the concept of sanctuary, an idea that has been with us for a long time. For centuries, individuals attempting to escape intolerable circumstances have been given respite in temples and churches. In our times, hospitals are being asked to perform this service, and often the admission ticket is a statement of suicidality. Such an admission is certainly not the best use of hospital resources. On the other hand, the hospital is often the only resource. In several parts of the United States, treatment programs are starting to reexplore the notion of providing sanctuary outside of a hospital setting to individuals whose functioning is compromised by overwhelming stress. Many systems now offer a range of placement options for patients in acute distress, not just a traditional hospital milieu. From our point of view, this development is a very positive one, because it may help us overcome some of the unintended side effects of hospitalization.

For now, respite care for suicidality is a legitimate use of the hospital and of a variety of step-down treatment options (e.g., 23-hour beds, crisis respite houses, and partial hospitals). At the time of admission, it is important that both staff and patient understand what is being done. The patient needs to agree that his or her current stress level is overwhelming and that the hospital can be useful by providing a safe place with plenty of help available for developing a plan for dealing with discomfort and dysphoria. The stay should be described as brief (no more than 48–72 hours) and as being the first step in dealing with the patient's stresses. This use affects the types of services provided to the patient. There is much less emphasis on diagnostic studies and medication trials and more emphasis on crisis support and problem solving. It is very helpful, as part of your strategy for continuing to reduce the level of stress, to have day hospital and residential services available as a logical, less-intense step in the treatment process.

Reshaping Suicidal Behavior: Planned Hospitalization

A third reason for hospitalization occurs when admissions are planned as part of a long-term shaping strategy, a strategy that can be helpful with *repetitiously suicidal individuals who have a history of multiple hospital admissions.* Almost always, hospital admissions have occurred on a *mental breakdown* basis. The strength of a planned admissions strategy is that it places future hospitalizations on a *health maintenance* basis. The technique is as follows: A review of previous records will determine the frequency of hospitalization. Future admissions are planned, generally at the end of a hospitalization, on the basis of this pattern. If admissions are occurring at 4-month intervals, the next admission should be planned for approximately 4 months after the end of the current hospitalization and for a duration somewhat less than the average length of stay of previous hospitalizations. The outpatient therapist can use this approach in several ways. One of the most important is to demonstrate to the patient that knowing that a period of respite is planned, he or she can tolerate emotional pain. Once the first planned admission is accomplished, the next admission should be negotiated for an interval longer than the usual period between hospitalizations. The hospital stay should be somewhat shorter than the previous stay. Repeating this process can result in less use of the hospital and can enable your patient to develop better coping skills.

> Ms. B is a 32-year-old woman who has been treated for approximately 10 years with both medications and psychotherapy for the diagnosis of "mixed personality." A planned admissions strategy was incorporated into her treatment approximately 3 years ago. Up until that point, the patient had been hospitalized approximately every 3 months, the length of stay being 3 days to 2 weeks each time. Hospitalization was planned for 3 months after discharge for a length of 5 days. During those interim 3 months, the patient reported distress on several occasions but agreed to wait for the planned hospitalization. At one point she appeared in the emergency department. She was asked to hold on until the date of the scheduled hospitalization. She was able to do so, and the planned admission went according to schedule. There was no crisis at the time of the first planned admission. During the 5-day stay, the patient focused on building a more competent social support network. The next planned hospitalization was then scheduled to take place 5 months later for a duration of 3 days. During the intervening 5 months, the patient went through several distressful emotional periods and once asked to be admitted. Other strategies were evoked (see Chapter 7, "Managing Suicidal Emergencies"), and Ms. B had less trouble agreeing to wait until the upcoming hospitalization. The third hospitalization was scheduled for 7 months after the second for a period of 3 days. As the date of the third hospitalization approached, the patient stated that she felt she did not need to be hospitalized this time and that it might interfere with her life. Her therapist argued about this decision with her, saying that the hospitalization was an important aspect of her health maintenance program. In the end, the patient agreed to the hospitalization, but only for 2 days. The next hospitalization was set for 10 months after the third, but this time the patient successfully argued that hospitalization was no longer a necessary part of her treatment plan.

Targets for a Short-Term Hospital Stay

Table 8–1 lists seven treatment targets for the short-term hospital treatment of a suicidal patient. Unlike outpatient treatment, in which treatment targets might be sequenced over weeks or months, the short-term hospital stay requires activity in all target areas almost from the day of admission. The first target is probably the essence of psychiatric hospitalization: *start treatment of psychiatric disorders* as indicated. Psychiatric illness is painful. It can be disorienting, and it can certainly contribute to suicidality. The second point, *validate emotional pain,* is a reference to Chapter 5 ("Outpatient Interventions With Suicidal Patients") in which you begin reframing the pain using the technique of the three *I*s: the pain is inescapable, intolerable, and interminable. In the hospital, it is most important to empathize with the patient's sense of emotional pain and desperation. After all, people do not enter a psychiatric hospital because life is going well. It is important to agree with the individual that he or she is suffering and to convey your understanding of that suffering. Reviewing the pain from the three-*I*s point of view will provide your patient with the acceptance and value problem-solving framework outlined in this book. The goals of the short-term stay are to identify problematic situations, learn to tolerate associated emotional discomfort, and begin to solve problems in ways that do not involve suicidal and self-destructive behavior. You may not be in a position to finish this process, but you can get it off to a very powerful start.

Table 8–1. Seven treatment targets for a short-term hospital stay

1. Start treatment for psychiatric disorders if indicated.
2. Validate emotional pain and destabilize the three *I*s.
3. Discuss and address the patient's ambivalence.
4. Provide encouragement on a regular basis.
5. Develop small-scale positive action plans.
6. Integrate the outpatient treatment plan and provider.
7. Evaluate and mobilize the social support network.

Consider offering specific skills training in various areas that might be beneficial to almost any psychiatric patient but are particularly pertinent for suicidal patients: problem-solving skills, mindfulness and acceptance, interpersonal skills, and self-directed behavior change skills. This work is most important, because it will set the stage for both further inpatient activities and the structure of treatment after discharge.

Ambivalence must be addressed with any suicidal individual: One part wants to live, one part wants to die. An excellent tool for exploring ambivalence is the Reasons for Living Inventory (Appendix C). The factors derived from this instrument (i.e., survival and coping beliefs, responsibility to family, child-related concerns, fear of suicide, fear of social disapproval, and moral objections) can provide a focus for a discussion of the positive side of ambivalence. This discussion of ambivalence will provide a context to move to initial work in problem solving, because it will show your patient that there are a range of feelings and a range of concerns with which to deal.

Providing encouragement has as much to do with attitude and demeanor as with what is said. The hospital staff needs to have confidence in the ward treatment scheme for suicidality and be confident that it is a process that will work. The organization of the team around a coherent plan is most important. Most inpatient services conduct daily team meetings to review progress and coordinate treatment. At each of these meetings, the question should be asked, Are we providing the proper encouragement? Suicidality is always capable of producing negative emotions in staff. A discussion about encouragement is an excellent way of getting at and dealing with these difficult provider feelings. Staff brainstorming on providing encouragement to a difficult patient generally produces both good ideas and needed attitude adjustment.

The *positive action plan* is a useful clinical alternative to the traditional *no-suicide contract*. In a no-suicide contract the patient agrees to exhibiting no suicidal behavior for a set period. The patient is asked to define a period in which he or she would be comfortable not engaging in suicidal behavior. Although useful in helping with pain tolerance, a contract like this does not allow the treatment team to use all the treatment modalities at their disposal. Converting the no-suicide contract to a positive action plan is more productive. A positive action plan is a way of negotiating a series of small constructive responses to suicidal ideation. These responses can be self-care, exercise, interpersonal contacts, spiritual activities, and the like. The focus is on developing tolerance for and diversion from emotional pain. These behaviors have the effect of helping the patient ride out an acute suicidal crisis. Like the no-suicide contract, a time limit should be negotiated. The time limit should be brief—hours to a few days. It is useful for staff to argue for a shorter period than the patient initially identifies while negotiating the plan. Define with the patient what specific actions are needed if an obstacle to implementation of the plan arises, and set up periodic check-ins to evaluate how the plan is working. Be absolutely certain that a staff member is present when the time frame for the positive action plan expires. At this point, the strategies are reviewed: Strategies that did not work are tossed out, new ones are instituted, and a new contract is written.

Outpatient treatment is always a factor in inpatient treatment. In this area breakdowns are both frequent and harmful. The inpatient and outpatient sectors are not separate delivery systems. They are part of a single continuum of care. There is no contest to see who "owns" the patient; treatment is designed to ensure that the patient receives comprehensive, coordinated care. From the first day of hospitalization, *the outpatient plan should be part of the inpatient plan and the discharge plan.* If the outpatient therapist is already involved, make sure he or she has input into the inpatient program. Seek the outpatient therapist's advice and solicit his or her ideas. If there is no ongoing outpatient treatment, it is the job of the inpatient team to initiate it.

The last point in the hospital plan is to *evaluate and mobilize the patient's social support network.* If at all possible, interview family and friends and evaluate their ability to provide competent social support. Family members and friends often would like to help, but they feel overwhelmed or burned out. Hearing them out and then offering instruction in how to offer competent social support is an important part of inpatient work. To mobilize the patient, consider using the various crisis strategies, such as the crisis card, described in Chapter 7 ("Managing Suicidal Emergencies"). This approach will help the patient learn to appropriately access social and community supports once discharged.

The Trouble With Discharge

Suicidal patients need coordinated and coherent care both across systems and among levels of care. A problem in moving between systems is the act of *discharge,* a term that is often taken to mean both release from care and severance of further responsibility. From the continuity of care point of view, far too many hospitals operate independently from outpatient treatment systems. Care is not finished just because the most intensive and expensive mode of treatment is no longer in effect. Arranging for outpatient treatment is a necessary part of the hospital plan, but *participating* in a system of care should be the goal of current planning. *Coordinated transfer planning* is a much better phrase for describing what needs to be done to move the patient from the hospital to the next step in treatment. The inpatient service should be part of a coordinated and interconnected network that provides various services within the context of a longer-term and coherent plan. This *integrated treatment and crisis response system,* the focus of the last part of this chapter, offers exciting and positive alternatives to the use of the hospital in treating suicidality.

Model Integrated Treatment and Crisis Response System

A major challenge facing the mental health system is to produce efficient and effective care for suicidal individuals. The use of hospitalization as a principal option for these people requires careful examination. We have already discussed the lack of efficacy: Hospitalization does not deliver on the assumption that it will reduce death by suicide. Furthermore, hospitalization is very expensive. Health care dollars are scarce, and dollars spent on hospitals are not available for development of better alternatives. Particularly in the public sector, it is absolutely essential to get the most out of each dollar spent. Patients stabilized in an inpatient environment are more likely to decompensate unless they receive continued outpatient support. Destabilization adds to the demand for crisis services and an increased demand for hospital care. If the dollars remain the same and hospital care increases, the only result can be further reduction in outpatient resources. The mental health system cannot afford this downward spiral. Crisis management in general and the treatment of suicidality in particular suffer. Hospital care is a precious and expensive resource and must be reserved for people who truly need it. An array of less-expensive, more-efficient, nonhospital alternatives must be developed. To meet this need, independent elements must work together. Emergency centers, hospitals, and outpatient facilities need to vigorously attack the current barriers to effective long-term care. The work is not easy. There are philosophical, administrative, and legal impediments to be overcome. Each community will face a different challenge, and each state needs to review its civil commitment and other mental illness processes. What follows is an outline of an integrated, five-component system, a system that is within the grasp of many communities.

Component 1: An Emergency Center

An emergency center is a hospital-based facility. It offers acute care for a variety of trauma and illnesses and is an entry point to either the hospital or the outpatient clinic. Emergency psychiatry is a significant service in any such center, and mental health workers in this system deal with a great variety of difficulties. The complexity of the evaluations can be enormous, requiring input from several medical specialties. An example, and a common one, is contained in the workup that might be required for a person brought in by the police "found down" and "acting confused and psychotic." The evaluator needs to look for many things, including head trauma, psychotic illness, acute substance abuse, and innumerable medical conditions, such as thyroid dysfunction and diabetes. Has this person overdosed? Is this toxic condition deliberate (a suicide attempt) or an accident? Individuals in this condition are often unknown to the emergency evaluating staff, and no information about the medical or psychiatric history is available.

To evaluate this patient, psychiatric, general medical, and neurological assessments must be conducted. In addition, staff must scramble to find out as much as they can: Is this person in treatment anywhere? Can we tap into that database? Often this information is difficult to obtain, especially at night and on weekends. Needed history can be difficult to impossible to obtain from patients, especially if the psychiatric state and medical aftermath of a suicide attempt make effective interviewing impossible. At that point, if you know the patient's identity, you should have ready access to the facts about him or her. Emergency centers can be linked via computer with state hospitals, mental health centers, and other sources. The fact that most centers are not linked is a sad comment on our multifaceted inability to cooperate between systems, especially when it comes to addressing our pervasive medical and legal fears. The legitimate sticking point in information exchange is patient confidentiality. This problem is dealt with mechanically with computer safeguards. At the crucial level, the problem is dealt with by interagency agreements whereby each agency is part of a system dealing with the same people and their problems over time. Unless we all strive to develop these tools, case management comes to its limits of efficacy fairly quickly.

In addition to acquiring information quickly, a second and powerful case management tool in an emergency center is appointment authority. Too often, psychiatric patients leave emergency centers with at best a phone number to call. This wish-and-a-prayer approach to follow-up is not effective. What should happen, and is now technically feasible, is this: A patient is evaluated and observed in an emergency setting, and treatment is initiated. If outpatient follow-up is the next logical step, the patient is given an appointment with an identified clinician. Two things should happen before that appointment. First, the provider on the receiving end needs to have available, in advance, all the information obtained from the emergency center evaluation. Second, a case manager must work to get the patient to the appointment. This process can involve a range of action, from a phone call (most of us know how good dentists are at this) to picking up the patient and transporting him or her to the follow-up appointment.

Component 2: Twenty-Four-Hour Holding Beds

The "found down" suicidal patient in the example may well need a lot of work before a rational disposition from an emergency center can be made. A patient often is admitted to an inpatient unit (the expensive option) because the emergency center is busy, patients need to be moved on, and the workup is incomplete. Having 24-hour holding beds can often eliminate this need for admission. Tests can be run, information gathered, observations made, and response to treatment observed. Having a bed for the patient and a calendar day to work with are much more satisfactory than feeling pressure to get the patient "somewhere, anywhere" within a maximum of 4–6 hours.

Component 3: A Brief-Stay Inpatient Service

A psychiatric unit is a critical part of an integrated crisis system. We define *brief stay* as anywhere from 2 to 21 days. Let us take our "found down" patient and expand his case. Like many psychiatric patients, the patient has more than one thing wrong with him. In the emergency center we learn the following:

> The patient is 43 years old. Twenty years ago, he was given the diagnosis of schizophrenia. His case is being followed by a mental health center, but he has not been seen for 6 weeks. Antipsychotic medication has been prescribed, but the patient does not like the side effects and has been noncompliant. The patient is alcoholic and is participating in the mental health center's newly formed dual-diagnosis program. He has poorly controlled insulin-dependent diabetes. A year ago, the patient was knocked unconscious and robbed, and his behavior has been more erratic since then. A week ago, he was kicked out of his boardinghouse because of drunkenness.

The emergency center evaluation reveals an acutely psychotic man who is also intoxicated. He talks of needing to kill himself before "the demons" kill him. His diabetic state requires immediate management. After 6 hours, the staff has an adequate diagnostic picture, and medical and psychiatric treatments are started. It is clear this man needs hospitalization, and he is admitted.

But for how long is the patient admitted? His acute psychosis might be well on the way to resolution in 3–6 days, and his diabetes brought under control even more quickly. As with most patients, the patient's acute suicidal ideation will probably abate in 3–5 days. He might well be transferred to a nonhospital option at that point, or continued problems might necessitate more time in house. For many patients, even with the complexity noted in the example, the time in the hospital after a week of treatment is determined less by some absolute need to remain an inpatient and more by the quality of other options.

Component 4: A Crisis Residential Unit

We discussed earlier (see When Should You Hospitalize a Patient?) the need for sanctuary, for a sheltering, safe environment where an individual can be housed and cared for and obtain a respite from the overwhelming daily hassles of life. Our "found down" patient has improved both physically and mentally. However, he needs continued monitoring regarding his medication, a place to stay, and integration with his the intensive outpatient programs at his mental health clinic. As the psychosis resolves, suicidality becomes more clearly related to the patient's loss of shelter and uncontrolled addictive disorder. Problems have been identified, and problem-solving therapy is initiated. These needs can safely be met in a residential milieu.

Component 5: A Crisis Stabilization Outpatient Program

The suicidal patient in the example will have his crises resolved, and he will return to long-term treatment for his chronic illnesses. Some of the neuropsychological deficits found have been the result of the blow to his head. Rehabilitation from this injury has been added to the therapy regimens. Other patients, however, do not have a chronic illness. Their crises, including suicidality, can be dealt with in a 1- to 3-month crisis intervention clinic. Such a clinic consists of mental health personnel trained in individual, family, and group support and in crisis resolution techniques. Crisis case management has a major role in this clinic, lending a firm hand to establishing or reestablishing a comprehensive system of support. Equally important is an understanding of the brief and judicious use of medications, especially when suicidal potential is involved.

Keep All the Doors Open

If an integrated system is to live up to its name, the suicidal patient must be able to move easily between components. Each part of the system has an unlocked door to every other part. *Movement is not failure.* It is based on clinical appropriateness. Inpatient services provide the most intensive diagnosis, observations, and treatment. Outpatient services deliver definitive therapy and integrate patients back into the community. Residential services are of intermediate intensity and provide sanctuary. Each component can function best knowing the other components are available. For example, staff members in an acute residential setting, if they have immediate hospital backup, will be much more comfortable taking a suicidal patient who is a little better but still is in a state of some disrepair. The outpatient setting can use a residential setting in lieu of the hospital. If information flows freely around the system, the only major impediment to movement through the doors is that peculiar medical paranoia: the fear of dumping.

Dumping—pushing the problem to someone else's bailiwick without concern for the patient's welfare—is the death of system development. Fight it like the plague. Feedback loops among all the components, which allow for open discussion about problems, will help. The key question for feedback discussion is, Are we working in the best interest of the patient? The second question is, Was transfer done to treat the patient, or was it done to treat our own difficulties, be they anger, a sense of failure, or job burnout? In addition to feedback, employ staff members who work both sides of the fence. Spending time, for example, in both the emergency center and in the residential setting will provide a perspective on how the two units work together that is far richer than working one place and speculating on how another place functions. In an integrated system, it is not us or them. It is all of us.

Helpful Hints

- Do not rely solely on the inpatient unit to treat suicidality; hospitals are overused and have not been shown to reduce death by suicide in any population.
- Hospital services are a critical component of an effective continuum of care for the suicidal patient, but only insofar as they integrate with the outpatient treatment plan and provider.
- When you use a hospital, make sure it is for the treatment of a psychiatric illness, for short-term sanctuary, or for reshaping suicidal behavior.
- Do not let your fear of malpractice litigation override your clinical judgment.
- An integrated crisis response system involves inpatient, step-down, and outpatient components in an all-doors-are-open model of service delivery.

Reference

Chiles JA, Strosahl KD, Ping ZY, et al: Depression, hopelessness, and suicidal behavior in Chinese and American psychiatric patients. Am J Psychiatry 146:339–344, 1989

Selected Readings

Bond GR, Witheridge TF, Wasmer D, et al: A comparison of two crisis housing alternatives to psychiatric hospitalization. Hosp Community Psychiatry 40:177–183, 1989

Chafetz L: Issues in emergency psychiatric research, in Emergency Psychiatry at the Crossroads: New Directions for Mental Health Services. Edited by Lipton F, Goldfinger S. San Francisco, CA, Jossey-Bass, 1985

Crammer JL: The special characteristics of suicide in hospital inpatients. Br J Psychiatry 145:460–476, 1984

Drye RC, Goulding RL, Goulding ME: No-suicide decision: patient monitoring of suicidal risk. Am J Psychiatry 130:171–174, 1973

Sunqvist-Stensmann UB: Suicides in close connection with psychiatric care: an analysis of 57 cases in a Swedish county. Acta Psychiatr Scand 76:15–20, 1987

9

Working With Special Populations

Substance-Abusing, Psychotic, Young, and Elderly Patients

The purpose of this book is to give you the tools needed to be effective in your assessment and treatment of the suicidal patient. To this end, we provide you with a structure for examining your own attitudes and philosophies about suicidality, a most necessary step in working in this challenging area. We then develop a series of comprehensive and specific techniques for treating the suicidal person. We realize treatment can occur in a variety of settings, and we have tailored this approach to the major settings: the family practitioner's office, the outpatient mental health clinic, and the psychiatric hospital. The approach outlined in this book can be helpful with almost any suicidal patient and in almost any setting. However, everyone is different, uniqueness abounds, and no amount of reading can fully prepare you for special situations.

In this chapter, we examine groups of patients who may call for the use of special techniques on your part. Included are the substance-abusing patient and the patient with a serious and persistent mental illness such as schizophrenia. Finally, we discuss how to address two age groups that pose special dilemmas in terms of managing their risk of suicidal behavior: adolescents and the elderly.

Medications and the Suicidal Patient: They Don't Work if You Don't Take Them, and They Don't Work if You Take Them All at Once

Many patients are treated with medications for their psychiatric illness. The three most common concerns in using medications to treat the suicidal patient are adherence (is your patient following the treatment regimen?), iatrogenesis (unintended negative effects on suicidality caused by the medicine), and the potential for overdose. Most commonly, patients are treated with antianxiety agents, antidepressants, or both. Less frequently they may be treated with antipsychotic medication or mood-stabilizing drugs. Mood stabilizers are used to treat bipolar disorder and are sometimes used to augment the efficacy of other psychiatric medications. In many chronically suicidal patients, mood stabilizers are used to lessen the patient's tendency toward emotional overarousal and impulsivity. As we review these medications, keep the following in mind.

First, understand how the medications might affect suicidality. When medications are effective, suicidality can be reduced as the problems produced by the mental illness diminish. However, when the medication is ineffective, or when troublesome side effects occur, suicidal behavior can increase. Know your medications, and use objective response criteria to determine whether they are being effective. As evidence-based treatment takes hold in the mental health field, response criteria (systematic and valid ways of determining whether a treatment is working) are coming into widespread use. You need to adjust your practice to begin incorporating empirically validated measurement techniques to track the progress your patient is making. We recommend that you take these measures at each contact with the patient to give you maximum sensitivity in determining what is changing for the better, what is not changing at all, and what is changing for the worse. A good source for such criteria used in major psychiatric disorders comes from the Texas Medication Algorithm Project (Chiles et al. 1999). In addition, if suicidality is in the picture, use one or more of the assessment devices in this book to track the patient's suicidality.

Second, when a patient is working with several health care providers, you need to understand the challenges and complexities that occur when a patient is working with two clinicians—one who is prescribing medications and the other who is delivering psychotherapy. In general, unless you are also providing both medicine and psychotherapy, the person responsible for the patient's overall treatment plan should be the psychotherapist. The therapist is in charge because medicines alone are insufficient treatment of patients with problem-solving styles that include suicidal behavior. The two care providers need to engage in a cooperative, rather than competitive, approach to treating the patient. Remember, when two providers start to compete for "ownership" of the patient, there is no winner, and ultimately the patient becomes a big loser.

Third, you need to become aware of the possible pitfalls associated with polymedication regimens, especially with repetitiously suicidal patients. Patients with chronic treatment-resistant problems such as suicidality can attract drugs like lightning rods. The sense of impotence that can develop in the provider often drives well-intended but clinically ineffective medication management regimens. Drugs can be useful in combinations, and patients at times benefit from two or more psychoactive medications. However, too many pills can be both psychologically and physically harmful. An approach to multi-medication regimens is described later (see Polymedication Regimens).

Antianxiety Agents

For several decades benzodiazepines have been the medications of choice for treating anxiety and agitation because of their positive impact on physiological overarousal. Benzodiazepines offer a major safety advantage over the medications they have replaced (barbiturates for the most part). Lethal overdoses are extremely uncommon. As a class, benzodiazepines have been a major advance in the medical pharmacopoeia. Outside of psychiatry, benzodiazepines are used effectively in a variety of neurological and general medical conditions. However, these agents present several major problems: They tend to be overused; they are not prescribed on a fixed daily schedule but instead are taken "prn"; they are often prescribed without an adequate monitoring plan; and they tend to be used too long. Overuse stems from the prescription of these medications as a quick fix for a potpourri of symptoms, such as poor sleep hygiene, excessive caffeine intake, and poor problem-solving skills. When a benzodiazepine is used to help a suicidal patient experiencing heightened levels of anxiety and agitation, a good general plan is to prescribe the drug at a dosage that provides short-term relief and to institute treatment that addresses the causes of the emotional difficulties. Many providers fall into the habit of letting patients decide when to use the medicine rather than setting up a plan of fixed daily doses. The as-needed model tends to lead to the use of very short-acting agents rather than longer-acting agents. The advantage of longer-acting agents is that they may have less abuse potential. Our clinical experience has shown that use of longer-acting agents breeds less psychological dependence. The patient is not allowed to make a quick association between popping a pill and rather immediately feeling significant distress reduction. For some patients taking short-acting medicines, a fast-acting chemical solution to problems will create a great deal less interest in developing the long-term problem-solving skills needed to build a more effective approach to life.

Our philosophy is to use an acute treatment approach with benzodiazepines: Use the medication for 2–6 weeks so that excessive emotional arousal does not interfere with the psychotherapeutic process, and then taper the drug to the point of discontinuation over several weeks. Longer use is justified in a small number of patients (those with chronic, severe anxiety complaints), but it can result in physical dependence and tolerance. Know the indications for long-term use, and document these indications in your chart notes if you prescribe a medication for longer than 3 months. The discontinuance of benzodiazepines can produce a variety of withdrawal symptoms, seizures being the most worrisome. In addition, some individuals who stop taking benzodiazepines experience, often several days later, rebound anxiety or rebound insomnia. In a suicidal individual, all of these phenomena can lead to increased dysphoria, agitation, and increased potential for suicidal behavior. When you are working with a patient who has been taking benzodiazepines for a considerable time, a good strategy is to set up a structured, gradual withdrawal program that may include the use of adjunctive medication. Remember, withdrawal symptoms from benzodiazepines can be similar to, and just as complex as, withdrawal symptoms from barbiturates or alcohol. Managing these phenomena can be tricky. If you are not familiar with these procedures, you need to consult with a colleague for this necessary treatment.

Antidepressant Medications

Antidepressants are a diverse class of drugs that have undergone a great deal of refinement since the early 1980s. The newer agents, represented mainly by the selective serotonin reuptake inhibitors (SSRIs), are no more effective than the older agents for treating depression but have a different side-effect profile, are generally easier to dose, and have much less lethal overdose potential. Monoamine oxidase inhibitors and tricyclic antidepressants both were developed in the 1950s, and both remain in use. Both types of drugs can be more effective, in some patients, than the newer agents. The side-effect profile of tricyclic antidepressants and monoamine oxidase inhibitors can cause adherence problems. However, a more serious problem is the overdose potential of these drugs. Because of the potential cardiovascular toxicity of both these classes of medication, a 2-week or even 1-week supply can be lethal. Often, because patients cannot be seen at more frequent intervals, these medications are prescribed for 30 days or more.

There are three concerns in the use of antidepressants to treat suicidal patients. *First, it is important to verify the diagnosis of depression.* As we have emphasized repeatedly, suicidality per se is not a sufficient condition for the diagnosis of depressive disorder, and there is no firm evidence that antidepressant medication is helpful with suicidality per se. Do not diagnose depressive disorder without using adequate criteria (American Psychiatric Association 2000). Do not assume that suicidal thoughts or actions per se justify this diagnosis. When the diagnosis turns out to be incorrect, the medical treatment has little chance of working and leaves your patient expecting a positive change that will not occur. This failed expectation runs the risk of increasing the patient's suicidality.

Second, if antidepressants are indicated, make sure the number of pills in the bottle makes up less than a lethal dose. For SSRIs, lethal dosing is not much of a problem—most individuals would need to take a number of months' supply to get into serious trouble. For tricyclic antidepressants, staying below lethal dose generally means administering 1- to 2-week prescriptions, keeping the total amount available less than 1,500–2,000 mg. Work with pharmacies to promote this plan. For example, you can write four 1-week prescriptions, dated to cover a month, rather than writing one prescription for the entire period. If this method proves difficult, family members or friends can be recruited to help keep your patient supplied with a reasonable amount of medication.

The problem with these management techniques is that although they promote safety, they also can emphasize passivity and dependence. Therefore it is important to work to gradually increase a sense of competency and security in self-managing medication. For example, you should rehearse ways in which your patient can take the initiative in discussing with the pharmacist ways of obtaining smaller prescriptions more frequently. Of course, patients will always be able to hoard medication, increasing the risk that if they do overdose, the results will be fatal. However, dealing with the total available dose as a treatment issue may well make hoarding less likely.

Another technique is, unfortunately, not readily available in the United States. This method involves packaging medication in individual wrappings. Over-the-counter medications are frequently dispensed this way. Many patients who overdose do so impulsively. The person is angry or upset and often is consuming alcohol. There is very little lead time, sometimes just a matter of a few minutes, between when the person decides to overdose and ingests the medication. Most of the pills in the bottle usually are consumed, and the person usually assumes the act of taking the pills will be lethal. The situation would be quite different if the patient were to have a long string of individually packaged pills. Unwrapping each pill might interfere with the impulsivity of the moment and make the situation safer.

A third potentially troublesome aspect of prescribing antidepressants, particularly the SSRI class of medicines, is the possibility that these drugs may have an iatrogenic effect on suicidality in certain populations. In the early 1990s there were scattered anecdotal reports linking use of an SSRI to increased suicidality. The pharmaceutical industry examined this connection in a number of data reanalyses and reported finding no evidence of any such connection for any SSRI that was studied. In 2003, however, researchers secured these original data sets under the Freedom of Information Act and reanalyzed the data (Healy 2003). The conclusion of the reanalysis was that there is a statistically significant association between the use of an SSRI and increased suicidality, particularly among adolescents.

There was a confound in the reanalyses of SSRIs. The original studies from which the data were taken excluded patients with any form of current or recent suicidal behavior and patients with potentially suicide-enhancing factors, such as drug or alcohol use and physical illness. Thus, the base rates of suicidal behavior were low. To the best of our knowledge, no studies of antidepressant medication have included actively suicidal depressed individuals and used suicidal behaviors as outcome measures. In addition, if more studies and reanalyses are forthcoming, keep in mind that antidepressants are a diverse group of drugs both kinetically and dynamically. Almost all these medications have effects on multiple neurotransmitters, some much more than others. For example, an increase in suicidality might be associated with an increase in agitation, which might be a product of the neurological side effect akathisia. Akathisia is generally believed to be a dopamine-modulated problem. Accordingly, this side effect is likely to be seen in the profile of some antidepressants but not others. Keep abreast of developments in this area, but do not assume that what is true for one antidepressant is true for another. In other words, do not throw the baby out with the bath water.

There is cause for concern. In the spring of 2003, both the U.S. Food and Drug Administration (FDA) and its counterpart in Great Britain issued a warning letter against using paroxetine (Paxil, Seroxat) in the treatment of children owing to increased risk of suicidal behavior. For the same reason, a warning has been issued against using venlafaxine (Effexor) to treat children. In March 2004, the FDA issued a warning on worsening depression and suicidality in patients being treated with certain antidepressants. Clinicians prescribing antidepressants should obtain this warning (www.fda.gov) and become familiar with its contents. We advise you to be very conscious of the potential for escalating suicidality among patients who have started treatment with an antidepressant and to follow the story as it evolves.

Antipsychotic Medications

Antipsychotic medications are a necessary ingredient in treating psychotic illness but can have untoward effects on a suicidal patient. *Some antipsychotics, particularly the first-generation ones, in addition to overdose concerns, have a side-effect profile that can aggravate suicidality.* Specifically, first-generation antipsychotics are associated with substantial risk of inducing neurological side effects. The most common side effects are known as *extrapyramidal symptoms*. One extrapyramidal symptom is akathisia, which is best described as an overwhelming desire to stay in motion, a constant and uncomfortable restlessness, and an inability to sit still. People experiencing this side effect can have a sustained and terrifying experience. Undiagnosed and untreated, akathisia has been specifically described in suicide notes as a cause of the patient's deadly behavior. This effect has occurred with use of these medications to treat a psychotic illness, but it also has occurred when patients have been given this class of drug for other indications (e.g., nausea and vomiting). A second extrapyramidal symptom that can be quite uncomfortable and is related to increasing suicidality is akinesia, which is difficulty initiating movement. As a chronic side effect, akinesia gives many patients a blunted and unresponsive physiognomy. Facial muscles do not work well, arms do not swing normally during walking, and the person looks stilted and odd. The overall effect can be medication-enhanced difficulties with communication and resulting social isolation. If not diagnosed and adequately addressed, both of these side effects can be instrumental in producing suicidality.

Second-generation antipsychotics are a significant pharmacological advance. They may offer better treatment of some of the severe symptoms of schizophrenia, particularly negative symptoms and some aspects of cognitive impairment, and their different side-effect profile (compared with that of first-generation drugs) offers advantages. Second-generation antipsychotics are less likely to produce akathisia and akinesia, lessening at least that risk of suicide. Be aware, however, that the metabolic side effects of some of these newer agents may make matters worse for your suicidal patient. We are particularly concerned with the onset of type 2 diabetes—diabetes has long been associated with increased risk of depression—and with excessive weight gain and its adverse effects on self-esteem.

Among the antipsychotics, clozapine, generally viewed in the United States as a third-line intervention in schizophrenia, was shown in a large double-blind study (Meltzer et al. 2003) to have significantly better effects than olanzapine on reducing both suicidal ideation and suicide attempts in patients with schizophrenia. The authors of the study are to be commended. To the best of our knowledge, the study was the only well-designed, prospective medication trial that included suicidal individuals and examined those particular behaviors.

Mood-Stabilizing Medications

Mood stabilization describes an effect, most usually sought in bipolar disorder, rather than a particular class of medication. Lithium, the standard of care, is the first of the mood stabilizers. Medications considered comparable to lithium include valproate, olanzapine, and possibly carbamazepine. There are clinical accounts of the use of a number of the newer anticonvulsant and second-generation antipsychotic medications for various aspects of mood stabilization, and some of these drugs are under investigation to determine whether mood stabilization is an indication of use. A discussion of each drug is beyond the scope of this book. If you use these medications, know them individually, and for use of these agents with a suicidal patient, follow the guidelines given later in this chapter (see later section, Polymedication Regimens).

Lithium deserves a special note. Lithium is the only pharmacological agent that has shown consistent positive effects on suicide rates over multiple studies. We laud the prospective clozapine study (Meltzer et al. 2003) but note that that effect was on nonlethal behaviors. Lithium, used primarily to treat patients with bipolar disorder, has a positive effect on the rate of death by suicide in that group of patients. Tondo et al. (2001) offer a good review of these studies.

Polymedication Regimens

Clinicians are increasingly aware that patients can have more than one psychiatric diagnosis, each requiring treatment. In addition, with the advent of new and more sophisticated medications in almost every drug class, a variety of augmentation strategies—coupled with a perception that each symptom can be individually targeted by a particular drug—has often led to the use of several medications at once in treating a patient with a single psychiatric illness. In general, the more numerous a patient's symptoms, the more likely it is he or she is taking multiple drugs. As a moderately extreme example, a patient with the diagnosis of bipolar disorder and borderline personality disorder may well be taking a combination such as lithium, valproic acid, haloperidol, lorazepam, benztropine, and propranolol to cover an array of symptoms and side effects.

The judicious use of multiple medications certainly has a place in modern psychiatry, but dangers do arise. We note them here because it is not unusual to find a suicidal person taking several different drugs, especially if he or she has made several suicide attempts and if he or she has several different psychiatric diagnoses.

First, some patients are exposed to polymedication regimens because health care information is not being shared among providers and distribution points. Several physicians may have prescribed medication, each not knowing of the other's involvement. One of us (J.A.C.) looked at the medications being prescribed for approximately 600 psychiatric patients by other clinics in a large county hospital and found that 22 patients were being given psychoactive medications (either antianxiety or antidepressant agents) by these clinic physicians. In most of these cases, these medications were not recorded in the psychiatry chart. The information became available only when the hospital opened up its integrated pharmacy database (if you have access to one of these databases, check your patients through it). Another irrational process is continuing medications after the prescribing physician quits the case. Some physicians have an unfortunate tendency to add new medications but not subtract old ones. Some pharmacies continue refills indefinitely. One of us (J.A.C.) treated a distressing case of tardive dyskinesia that emerged after a 48-year-old woman had been treated with thioridazine for 15 years. This medicine, at 50 mg per night, had originally been prescribed for insomnia. The treating physician died, and the local drugstore continued to refill the prescription for years. The woman saw other physicians during this time for treatment of depression. None of them was aware of the ongoing antipsychotic treatment. Make sure when you become involved in the care of a patient that polypharmacy has been arrived at by a rational process.

A second problem with polymedication regimens is that they have a multiplicative impact on side effects. An informal rule is that side-effect potential squares with each medication addition. Two pills have 4 times the side-effect potential of one pill, three pills have 9 times the potential, four pills have 16 times the potential, and five pills (this is the point where you really need to start thinking things over) have 25 times the side-effect potential of one pill. In addition to side effects increasing rapidly in numbers, individual side effects can be made worse. For example, a patient taking several drugs with anticholinergic properties can experience significant constipation, a condition sometimes not reported and often not asked about.

Third, medications can interact with the pharmacokinetic properties of one another in a variety of ways that create swings in blood levels that can lead to both adverse events and ineffective levels of the medication. You must understand the pharmacokinetics and pharmacodynamics of the medications you prescribe to be in the best position to avoid or treat these interactive problems. However, all your knowledge ceases to be of much use when three or more drugs are being used at once. At this point, drug therapy can become so complex that no one knows what is going on or what might happen.

The following are a few rules that will help to keep you out of trouble with polypharmacy regimens:

1. Have a good reason for adding a drug, and document it.
2. Use a medication in sufficient dose and for a sufficient length of time to determine whether it is working. Do not add a medicine until you are sure the patient has taken the first one as prescribed, at a therapeutic level, and for long enough to verify that it does or does not produce a benefit.
3. Use response criteria to gauge effectiveness. Stop the medication if it is not working. If possible, discontinue the drug in a tapering manner to avoid adverse rebound or withdrawal phenomena.
4. Keep your patient as active as possible in sizing up the effect of the new medication (e.g., include your patient's assessment in the clinical trial process).
5. Change only one drug at a time when possible. It is difficult enough to gauge the effect of the addition or subtraction of one drug, let alone two or three.
6. Be cautious about adding medicines simply because a suicidal crisis is present. As in our philosophy about therapy, the recurrence of suicidality does not mean that treatment is failing.

One last rule: You have the three *I*s for evaluating problems associated with suicidality. The following are the three *A*s for evaluating medications:

- *Appropriateness:* Is the diagnosis correct? Is the drug the correct treatment of the diagnosis? With polypharmacy, is there a legitimate reason for each medication? Is the medication effective? Are appropriate response criteria being used?

- *Adherence:* Is your patient taking the medication as directed? If not, why not?
- *Adverse effects:* Know the adverse effects of a drug. Ask about them. Early recognition of side effects generally makes them much easier to manage.

Case Management in Microcosm: The Prescribing Physician–Therapist–Patient Triangle

A number of patients see both a psychotherapist and a pharmacotherapist. In Medications and the Suicidal Patient, we describe a philosophy that emphasizes coordination, rather than competition, between providers. At its best, the triangle of care consisting of prescribing physician, therapist, and patient provides a complete and well-coordinated treatment program infused with ideas from the perspectives of two providers. At worst, one provider, willingly or unwillingly, can be set against the other. Success in a triangular relationship is accomplished by a clear definition of roles and responsibilities and with agreements on types of treatment that are being applied. The patient should give informed consent to the treatments involved. Various clinic policies, including fees for both providers, should be made clear. Both providers should be explicit in how they handle emergencies and how coverage will be arranged when neither is available. The limits of protecting the patient's confidence between providers should be discussed, and a clear statement should be made that each provider will consult with the other on a regular basis. Both providers need to keep good written records.

A basic rule for establishing triangular arrangements is that neither provider should commit the other to a course of treatment. A patient should never be guaranteed that he or she will be given medication or a certain form of psychotherapy. A referral should always be something such as, "This might be a good idea; let's see what my colleague thinks." *A second rule is that the patient's treatment plan should integrate the goals of the pharmacotherapist and the psychotherapist.* In other words, both providers need to consciously attempt to form a unified treatment plan for the patient. Further information about integrating pharmacotherapy and psychotherapy is provided in Selected Readings. In most cases, medication plays an important, but secondary, role in the treatment of the suicidal patient. Thus, the provider in charge of the overall treatment plan should be the psychotherapist. *A final rule is that decisions about the ultimate goals of treatment should be the responsibility of the treating therapist.*

One of the more volatile and potentially destructive moments in the course of treatment occurs when one provider believes the treatment implemented by the other provider is not helping the patient. This scenario takes a variety of forms with which most practitioners are personally familiar and which may involve the practitioner's feeling that a therapy is groundless, wandering, or occurring so infrequently as to be hardly beneficial to the patient. The medical practitioner may begin to harbor beliefs regarding the therapist's competence to handle the difficulties imposed by the patient. At the same time, the patient may indicate a strong sense of rapport and caring for the therapist, making treatment efficacy an extremely sensitive issue to approach. Another common scenario is that the medical practitioner believes the therapist is advising the patient about how to use medications or is passively encouraging the patient to discontinue medication because the therapist believes the medications are not working. On the other hand, nonmedical therapists often experience frustration over the fact that medication regimens do not seem to be working but are nonetheless being continued by the medical practitioner. A more basic difficulty can involve suspicion about the value of medications in general in treating mental disorders. The therapist may be strongly opposed in principle to the use of any medication despite both the patient's request and data supporting use of the drug. Rather than put this agenda on the table, the therapist may subtly sabotage the patient's compliance and passively undermine the medical practitioner. In another scenario, the therapist senses that the interactions between the medical practitioner and the patient are for one reason or another undercutting the treatment being delivered by the therapist. The therapist may have assumed the patient is going to the medical practitioner for medications only and feels undermined when the medical practitioner gives the patient advice about how to deal with problems. The therapist perceives this advice as contradicting what is being promoted in therapy.

The solution to these troublesome situations is obvious: The two practitioners need to consult with each other regarding how the treatment is going and how the limits of professional responsibility are being met by each. Unfortunately, this professional interaction can be a difficult one to undertake. As a consequence, the interaction is frequently and easily avoided. Good practitioners need to see it as their ethical responsibility to negotiate these types of troubled waters. In general, the patient's welfare is at stake, even though the practitioners' egos may be on the line. Another troublesome aspect of this type of situation is that when a confrontation between colleagues does occur, the patient may be blamed for splitting the therapist and the medical practitioner. In other words, the patient is presented as manipulative as an explanation for a basic professional boundary disagreement between the therapist and the medical provider. Remember this point: *If no split exists between the two providers, there will be no splitting.*

Substance Abuse and Suicide: The Patient Who Is Left Out in the Cold

All health care providers are aware of the enormity of substance abuse problems. Whether you work in a general health care setting, a trauma center, or a mental health facility, many of your patients have the added impairment of substance abuse or dependency. This area is of particular concern in psychiatric medicine, in which mentally ill, chemically affected individuals are a large part of the treated population, especially in the public setting. The combined disorders usually cause severe impairment. All areas of functioning can be adversely affected, including family and social interactions, employment, and the ability to meet the basic needs of shelter and food. Drug and alcohol use disorders vary markedly, ranging from infrequent bouts of alcohol intoxication to the daily use of a number of substances. In many cases, it is not uncommon to find someone who is using marijuana, cocaine, and alcohol on a daily basis and who has a number of medical problems in addition to or because of substance abuse. Patients with substance use disorders are often difficult to treat, and a major component of that difficulty can be a lack of motivation for treatment and lack of compliance with treatment. There is extensive literature on the practical issues involved in rehabilitation and recovery from substance use disorders. Several references that we have found helpful appear in the Selected Readings at the end of this chapter. Our concern is that this population of patients is fraught with suicidality. The patients can be difficult to treat and can find themselves caught between agencies and finding no one to address the totality of their problems. A problem-solving approach can work with these individuals, but someone has to administer it.

A major difficulty in providing effective management of the substance-abusing suicidal patient is the reluctance to assume responsibility for care that affects both mental health and chemical dependency treatment systems. This distressingly common scenario is played out in the following way: The mental health clinician or the inpatient psychiatric unit refuses to work with the patient because of the continuation of substance abuse. The message is that the patient must get his or her substance abuse cleared up before mental health treatment can proceed. On the other side, the substance-abusing patient enters the chemical dependency treatment system, either an inpatient or outpatient program, and experiences suicidality. The patient is immediately discharged from that system with the message that the suicidality needs to be brought under control before chemical dependency treatment can be administered. Some authorities have suggested that the real answer for this dilemma is to create a third service-delivery system—the dually diagnosed patient treatment system. This approach seems to obscure the fact that both mental health and chemical dependency counselors are professionally responsible for diagnosing and treating the array of mental and substance abuse conditions associated with patients who seek care in either system. A mental health counselor needs a strong and sophisticated set of skills in diagnosing and treating substance abuse. A chemical dependency worker needs a good working knowledge of how to deal with suicidal behavior. Unfortunately, both of these disciplines have put too much energy into criticizing one another, a practice that does little to alleviate the fact that a large number of patients travel between the two systems and are not receiving comprehensive care. Remember, in any setting, it is your professional responsibility to become concerned with the diagnosis and treatment of conditions that are presented to you for care. Patients often do not do a very good job sorting themselves out according to our ideas on how to treat them. The accommodation is our responsibility, not theirs. Practitioners in the chemical dependency, mental health, and general health care systems need to be prepared for the issue of suicidality and concurrent substance abuse.

The Substance-Abusing Suicidal Patient

The *AIM* model describes three crucial steps you must follow in evaluating and treating a substance-abusing, suicidal patient:

- *A*: Ask and ask again about substance use.
- *I*: Integrate substance abuse into the problem-solving context of suicidal behavior.
- *M*: Manage—develop a crisis management plan for handling escalating suicidality due to substance abuse.

It is important to recognize that alcohol and drug abuse shares important functional similarities with suicidal behavior: Both suicide and substance abuse are ways of controlling or avoiding unpleasant emotional content, and both function as problem-solving behaviors. You can "check out" by trying to kill yourself, or you can do so by getting numbed out from a drug-induced high. Because they are "birds of a feather," there is a high association between drugs, alcohol, and suicidality. This association presents both a challenge and an opportunity in treatment. Left undetected, unintegrated, and unmanaged, substance abuse can unravel your best treatment plan. Detected, integrated and managed, episodes of substance abuse can be used to further the goals of treatment, much the way episodes of suicidality can.

The first step is to learn how to ask about substance abuse and then ask about it again. This diagnostic task can be complex. It is not only a question of remembering to ask. It is also a question of persistence, of getting across your desire to be helpful, and of learning how not to be defeated by denial. A colleague related the following story, which demonstrates the scope of the problem:

> A woman appeared at a university-based affective disorders clinic for treatment of depression and persistent suicidality. Because the facility was a teaching clinic, the woman was interviewed by medical students, residents, and faculty. Each time, with structured interview techniques, the woman was systematically asked about substance abuse. In every instance, she denied any difficulties. Over the course of a stormy year of treatment, the woman showed little response to medicines or psychotherapy. During this time she made several suicide attempts. At the end, she failed to keep several appointments, and her relationship with the clinic stopped. Approximately a year and a half after the woman's last visit, one of the physicians in the clinic came across a newspaper article about this woman. She was being interviewed about her successful recovery from severe cocaine addiction. In the interview, the woman talked about a decade-long addictive disorder and a successful treatment program she had been working in for 6 months. There was no mention in the interview of her year-long treatment for depression and suicidality.

The lesson from this story is to ask, ask again, and ask in different ways. If physical symptoms, laboratory tests, and reports from family and friends keep your index of suspicion high, keep inquiring. Persistence can sometimes pay off. An undiagnosed and untreated addiction problem will make treatment of any other problem, including suicidality, difficult. It is almost a prescription for treatment failure.

Ask about both the actual use of substances and the effects of substances. A good question, using alcohol as an example, is as follows: "How many days during the past month have you had a drink? On those days when you had a drink, how many drinks did you have?" A frequently used acronym for substance abuse is *CAGE,* which refers to four questions. *C* stands for *cut down:* "Have you ever tried to cut down on your substance use?" *A* stands for *annoyed:* "Have other people become annoyed with you about your substance use?" *G* stands for *guilty:* "Have you ever felt guilty about your substance abuse?" *E* stands for *eye opener:* "Have you ever used (this substance) the first thing in the morning to avoid withdrawal symptoms (i.e., an eye opener)?" A yes to any of these questions can indicate a problem.

The second step is to understand substance abuse in the context of your patient's suicidality. The presence of suicidality suggests that a tandem addictive disorder may be present. People who use suicidality as a means of problem solving often engage in binge eating, binge drinking, and various forms of substance abuse. When you are working with your patient, always try to figure out the role of alcohol, cocaine, marijuana, or anything else being abused in the context of the patient's suicidality. Does your patient view suicidality as a solution to the chronic addiction? Does the patient use drugs or alcohol to escape the emotional pain associated with daily hassles and major stresses? When you are using problem-solving therapy, the effects of substance use can be most detrimental. Just when your patient needs to be thinking most clearly, the use of drugs can adversely affect judgment, concentration, and ability to think things through and can cause the patient to become more impulsive. This combination can be deadly, as evidenced by the alcohol level recorded in many a coroner's report after suicide. In addition, when overdose is the method of suicide attempt, many drugs of abuse, especially alcohol, will potentiate the lethal effects of the overdosing medication, making the situation that much more deadly.

The third step is to deal with substance abuse in a crisis management plan. A common scenario is as follows: The person whom you are treating is in a problem situation, dealing with an interpersonal difficulty. The patient becomes frustrated and angry. He or she starts to drink to alleviate this emotional pain. The drinking persists, and suddenly, and usually very rapidly, the solution of suicide becomes real. At this moment, the patient will often grab a bottle of pills and take them with the intent of dying. Impulsivity is increased by alcohol and so is the potential lethality of the overdose substance. It is a bad situation. The crisis management plan needs to address this situation before it arises: *When you are thinking about suicide, "Do not drink! If you are drinking, stop!"*

Alcohol on Breath: AOB in the Clinic

What do you do when your substance-abusing, suicidal patient arrives for treatment intoxicated? Your biggest challenge is to use this event in a way that ultimately benefits the patient and at the same time avoids a destructive, treatment-ending showdown over whether the substance abuse will continue. You must do your best to maintain a relationship with an impaired patient. These moments can be a rare opportunity for accessing something your patient may be very reluctant to talk about: the desperation with which negative feelings are avoided. Do not cancel the session or ignore the circumstance. Rather, praise your patient for having the courage to bring such a problematic behavior directly into the treatment. When you use this technique, you are being philosophically consistent with the problem-solving approach to suicidal behavior, namely, that it is permissible to bring your problems into the therapeutic context without unhinging the therapy. The goal in this strategy is certainly not to reinforce drinking behavior. The goal is to get past the impairing effects of drug and alcohol consumption and to understand what your patient is experiencing during this impaired state. Alcohol disinhibits the expression of emotion and cognition. Although alcohol has a depressant quality, it is likely that much of the feeling and thinking expressed by your patient under the influence has a real and substantial independent life. It is your task to sort out what part of the intoxication is impulsive and temporary and what part is giving you a look at thoughts, feelings, and reactions that are integral to your patient's worldview. This process requires a rapport between you and your patient, and it requires you to adopt a nonconfrontational stance concerning alcohol and drug consumption. Approximately 50% of all suicide attempts occur in the context of alcohol or drug use, so it is quite likely that proceeding with the session will give you insight into the process by which your patient engages in suicidal behavior. A behavioral crisis protocol is easier to produce if you have a comprehensive view of the way that this behavior develops during an episode of alcohol or drug abuse.

Your patient may arrive at the session intoxicated *and* acutely suicidal. In this case, your task is to help the patient get through impulsive and potentially lethal moments until a clear head prevails. It is generally advisable to keep the patient in a safe setting or to send the patient home with a friend or family member with explicit instructions that that person should remain in the immediate vicinity until the intoxication has cleared. As always, the general philosophy is to use whatever your patient brings in a way that provides advantage to the patient. In this respect, it is sometimes helpful to call the patient back and conduct a debriefing about whether the episode of alcohol or drug use seemed to work in terms of improving or worsening both mood and general life outlook. The more you can use dysfunctional problem solving and connect it with the experience of lack of workability, the more leverage you will have in getting your patient to consider alternatives.

The Inpatient Substance Abuse Unit

The staff on an inpatient chemical dependency unit deals with problems somewhat different from those encountered in an outpatient chemical dependency setting. The chief task of inpatient treatment is to assist the patient in getting through withdrawal and into early stages of sobriety maintenance. Withdrawal can be associated with an increase in suicidality. It is often a difficult process and has both physical and psychological components. Withdrawal can create agitation, physical discomfort, and significant mood swings. Because withdrawal symptoms can persist in some people for 2 months or more, it is sometimes difficult to determine what the long-term psychological dysfunction is and what the short-term dysfunction due to drug withdrawal is. Most physical effects of addiction and withdrawal improve within 10–14 days, but both sleep difficulties and psychological discomfort can continue for some time and can influence your patient's behavior. Depression is often a major and complicated problem sustained by continuous substance abuse and, in many cases, exists before the substance abuse. Your patient may be dealing with a "double whammy": organically induced depression due to a stage of drug use (acute or chronic withdrawal, sustained use, or intoxication) combined with a preexisting tendency to be depressed. Add the agitation and physical discomfort often associated with drugs, and the stage is set for potentially lethal suicidal behavior.

Many substance-abusing patients have comorbid psychiatric conditions. These conditions include depression, anxiety, personality disorders, and schizophrenia, all of which are associated with suicidal potential. A psychiatric examination, including assessment of suicidality, should be performed with any patient who is admitted to a substance abuse unit. By all accounts, this population is at high risk of both completed and attempted suicide, and admission for detoxification is a particularly critical phase in management of the disorder. Staff members need to learn how to assess and manage suicidal potential, especially during intensive substance-abuse treatment. These processes are conducted with the same techniques used on a psychiatric inpatient service (see Chapter 8, "Hospitals and Suicidal Behavior"), and there is no reason to believe that applications of these strategies would be any less effective in a substance-abuse treatment facility. The task is to provide as much safety and security as possible while avoiding an invasive, nontherapeutic milieu. The unit should adopt policies and procedures that systematize the way in which suicidal behavior assessments are conducted. Appropriate attention should be paid to documenting and treating any psychiatric conditions that may further increase the patient's suicidality.

A clinically significant difference between many substance-abusing patients and their nonabusing counterparts is the potential for tremendous mood variability that occurs in the first 30 days of treatment following withdrawal. Suicides on detoxification units sometimes occur when the patient is reporting a positive and stabilized mood. Consider the following clinical example:

> One of us (K. S.) treated a patient who had both chronic suicidal ideation and a long history of almost daily intoxication. As therapy progressed, the patient's suicidality diminished, but the drinking behavior escalated and led the patient to accept placement for 30 days in an inpatient treatment program. At first, things seemed to be going quite well. After several days of acute withdrawal symptoms managed by medication, the patient's sensorium began to clear, and his affect improved. He began talking about looking forward to a life free of daily struggle to stay sober. He reestablished contacts with some

family members who had been alienated by his drinking. Two weeks into the treatment he had become a model patient, attending and participating in various group and individual activities. His affect was stable, and he started to plan for his eventual discharge. On the fifteenth day, the patient ate lunch with everyone, joked around, seemed to be in good spirits, mentioned that he needed to make a phone call to a family member, and excused himself. Fifteen minutes later he was found hanging by a bedsheet in his room and was pronounced dead at the scene.

We do not know what went through this patient's mind that led to his sudden decision to commit suicide. However, it is important to understand that microepisodes of extreme dysphoria can occur within the context of overall improvement and can occur quite rapidly. The suicidal situation may happen in a matter of seconds or minutes, when the patient experiences a sudden devastating decline in mood and resorts to lethal behavior. The detoxifying patient's positive mood is not the result of a decision to commit suicide that has been made but not revealed. Rather, the suicidality seems to be linked to the rapid and unpredictable change in mood often associated with alcohol or drug withdrawal. Staff members need to be alert to these potential mood changes and specifically discuss the possibility with the patient at the onset of detoxification. Observation is not enough. Your patient needs to be asked frequently about mood and told repeatedly about the *necessity* of reporting any significant mood changes. Do not forget to repeat this process as the time for discharge back into the real, and often troubled, world approaches. Mood changes in this period may be pronounced, be missed, and be fatal.

The Special Case of Schizophrenia

Individuals with schizophrenia are prone to suicidal behavior in all its forms. Often their illness interferes with their relationships and their ability to concentrate and think clearly. From our point of view, their tools for problem solving are impaired. Isolation is a fact of life for many individuals with schizophrenia. Many of these people are homeless, and many seem likely to remain homeless. In this harsh atmosphere, many of these people are not likely to have access to treatment, or they have trouble being adherent with treatment when it is available. In addition, as we have learned from projects such as the Patient Outcomes Research Team and the Texas Medication Algorithm Project, many clinics do not offer adequate treatment to patients who do seek help. These individuals often have more than one illness. This tendency toward comorbidity encompasses both psychiatric and general medical disease. Substance abuse has become a rampant problem among patients with schizophrenia. All of these factors can produce a life full of stress and a sea of daily troubles far beyond that of the rest of us. With so many problems, the deficiency in the tools needed to deal with them, and the lack of adequate resources in many clinics, it is little wonder that suicidality is a major concern among patients with schizophrenia.

Individuals with schizophrenia are the core group of the chronic mentally ill. The lifetime rate of suicide in this population may be as high as 10%. One-third to one-half of individuals with schizophrenia have made a suicide attempt, and suicidal ideation is so common as to be nearly ubiquitous. Many individuals with this illness have only a partial response to treatment. The good news is that better treatments are available, and we can hope that in the near future improvements in negative symptoms and cognitions will be the expected outcome for all patients with this illness. With the reintroduction of clozapine in the United States, with the development of the second generation of medications for schizophrenia, and with additional unique antipsychotic medications under investigation, improvements are being seen in patients with schizophrenia that would have been judged quite improbable 10 years ago. If you are a clinician working with schizophrenia patients, part of your job from this point on is to keep the patients going until new and better therapies are widely available. Suicidality is one of the risk factors with which you must deal. What follows are special techniques that should help you in this work.

First, pay meticulous attention to the assessment of suicidality. Ask about suicidality and always remember this rule: The answers, not the affect, are important. Apathy and indifference are symptoms of schizophrenia. Answers to your questions will often be given in a flat and monosyllabic way. Someone with this flat affect is a far cry from an anxious, depressed, or despairing individual who talks about suicide and whose affect adds to the impact of what is said. Do not allow the lack of affect to subtract from the importance of what an individual with schizophrenia is saying. Lack of affect does not mean lack of risk. It is *what* is being said, not how it is being said.

Second, remember that an unintended effect of antipsychotic medications is an increase in suicidality. The side-effect profile of some these medications can produce a high level of discomfort. It is a terrible mistake to view these symptoms as an indication of increasing severity of schizophrenia and to treat them with even more medication. If you are not comfortable with the intricacies of medication management in schizophrenia, be sure you work with someone who is. In addition, remember that abrupt discontinuation of antipsychotic medication can produce both a number of withdrawal difficulties and an exacerbation of psychosis. Always taper administration when you are stopping a drug, and follow accepted guidelines for switching from one drug to another. Abrupt cessation of an antipsychotic medication is justified only when you are dealing with a serious side effect such as agranulocytosis.

Third, use the problem-solving approach to suicidality with schizophrenic patients, and be especially practical about it. Make every effort to involve supportive persons either from within the family or without. Carefully understand past episodes of suicidality, particularly as they relate to phase of illness. Talk over what happened earlier, and develop management strategies for possible recurrence.

The Young: Working With Suicidal Children and Adolescents

We seem to be facing a growing epidemic of suicidality in our young people. The pervasiveness of suicidal behavior is illustrated by the 1997 National Youth Risk Survey, which showed that approximately one in five youths younger than 18 years had experienced serious suicidal ideation. Sadly, an additional 7% made a suicide attempt. The statistics from the 2002 National Youth Risk Survey are an even greater cause for concern. In one upscale section of a central Michigan town, 29% of youths younger than 18 years admitted to serious suicidal behavior in the past year. Although rates of suicide in the 15- to 19-year age group remain lower than in the 20- to 24-year group, they have been rising all the same. What is particularly distressing is that the rates of nonfatal suicidal behavior and self-mutilation seem to be skyrocketing at the same time various suicide prevention initiatives have been launched in the nation's school systems. Programs such as peer helpers do not seem to have had the desired effect of forestalling fatal and nonfatal suicidal behavior in this age group. If these trends continue, practicing clinicians will have to become extremely adept at handling more and more suicidal adolescents.

It is hard to know what to make of suicidality in prepubertal children. Completed suicide is extremely rare in this group, even though both thoughts of death and thoughts of suicide are reported. There seems to be something about cognitive immaturity that protects against suicide. With adolescence, particularly middle to late adolescence, suicidality can become a significant issue. There are many similarities between the suicidality that occurs in adolescence and that which occurs in adulthood. The model presented in this book has been successfully applied with adolescents. The sole caveat is that attention must be paid to family-based matters. Suicidal adolescents often experience significant turmoil in their families. The turmoil starts in childhood and does not stabilize during adolescence. Adolescence produces further instability, and from all this comes suicidality.

An Adolescent Suicidal Behavior Scenario

A frequently seen adolescent suicidal behavior scenario starts with a long-term identity as a problem child. In early to middle adolescence, the usual mild to moderate troubles that arise from rearing a teenager escalate. The teenager can be the cause of family conflict and the destroyer of family harmony. Parents may block out the adolescent, pretend indifference, and view the teenager as somehow expendable. In some families, one or both parents may directly suggest that the family would be better off if the teenager were dead. The net effect is that family attention is increasingly contingent on extreme behavior. When problems are discussed, unrealistic and immediate solutions are emphasized over practical ones. Parents can assume that the adolescent is willfully acting bad rather than lacking the tools to change his or her behavior. In this scenario, suicide can easily take on a positive valence.

When coupled with ongoing family conflict, other forms of instability can fan the fire. The instability can include changes in residence, school troubles, loss of relationships (including parental divorce), and the phenomenon of *fractured romance*. Fractured romance is a situation in which a troubled adolescent has essentially put all his or her eggs in one basket. Another individual is seen as all-important and imbued with unique powers to bring stability into the teenager's life. When this relationship falls apart, as it often does, a major negative emotional event ensues. The potentially suicidal adolescent already has difficulty tolerating emotional distress, and the new distress seems overwhelmingly intense and persistent. When the distress is coupled with an impulsive behavioral style (actions speak louder than words) and alcohol or drug abuse, a scenario for suicidal behavior has been produced.

Family Evaluation Is a Must: Therapy May Be a Bust

Family dynamics can play a major role in adolescent suicidal behavior. Table 9–1 lists some of the more common features found in studies of families in which suicidal behavior has occurred. Not all families containing a suicidal adolescent are dysfunctional, but some certainly are. In any case, a family evaluation will be helpful and will guide your decision making.

In the face of family dysfunction, you can, at one end, engage the family in treatment to build cohesion and learn group problem solving or, at the other end, help extricate the adolescent from the system. There is not much evidence one way or the other concerning the utility of family therapy per se with the suicidal adolescent. Some families strongly resist change and cannot, despite strenuous effort, be enlisted as viable support for their teenage member. The dynamics of some families actively undermine the process of treating an adolescent using the problem-solving model. In a family environment that emphasizes action over words, models alcohol and drug abuse, and demands instant change, it is very difficult for an adolescent to effectively practice problem-solving skills. Much of the work done in this type of circumstance is to prepare the adolescent for early emancipation from the system. This preparation frequently involves teaching your patient limit setting and conflict resolution skills as well as specific anger management strategies. Sometimes the most important steps involve lining up an alternative residence with the parent of a willing friend or supporting the adolescent's effort to move in with a relative who is more supportive. The intent is not to break up families but to acknowledge that there is a power differential in family systems and that the adolescent is typically at the bottom of the totem pole. In effect, moving to the level at which the adolescent lives is a form of problem-solving behavior. This instance may be one of the few in which escaping or avoiding a stressful environment is a healthy maneuver.

Our overall recommendation in the treatment of teenagers is to pursue the approaches toward suicidality outlined in this book. Dysfunctional family behaviors need to be addressed. A family evaluation should always be done, and, if possible, the family should be in that part of treatment designed to put

Table 9–1.   The suicidal behavior–prone family

A. Chronic difficulties

   1. Long-term hostility, insecurity, asocial conduct, economic distress, alcohol abuse, troubled marriages

B. Active parent-child conflict

   1. Verbal, physical, sexual abuse
   2. Families report "daily fights"

C. Social characteristics

   1. Socially isolated
   2. May be very mobile
   3. Constant life stress (sea of troubles)

D. Fixed roles—rigid style

   1. Scapegoated child, parentified child, expendable child
   2. Position maintained by intolerance for loss and separation; change not possible, only escape

E. Loss of parent

   1. Divorce, desertion, separation
   2. Physically and emotionally distant parents are very demanding during infrequent contacts

F. Communication

   1. Ineffective
   2. Language has little problem-solving value—"spare the rod, spoil the child"
   3. Parents align to shut out children, yet will bolster child's negative stance toward outside intervention
   4. "Scapegoating" to "solve" parental conflict
   5. Basic belief that people can change by force of will; they do not have to learn anything new

together a competent social support system. Working with suicidal adolescents can provide a maximum challenge to a provider's skills. Some parents can seem persistently contentious, uncooperative, and angry. Skill in knowing when to and when not to deal with families is an essential prerequisite for working with adolescents.

There is one final point to keep in mind when treating adolescents. It is quite important to be constantly on the lookout for actions and thoughts that can be given a positive connotation. Negative self-esteem is a significant and nearly universal problem for this group. An unresponsive teenager can be praised for coming and being in the session, even when the task at hand seems overwhelming. Similarly, the adolescent whose fury at parents is massive can be praised for loyalty, as in the following example: "Your loyalty to your family is quite strong. Your anger, pain, and frustration are very evident, but somehow you've been able to stick with them. You are hanging in there every day, fighting to get them to change. Where do you get the strength?" A good rule to keep in mind is that the only time you have a reason to get upset is when your patient does not show up for treatment. When you are working together, your most important job is to find the positive side of ambivalence and the hidden strengths that will improve self-esteem.

The Forgotten Many: Suicidal Behavior in the Elderly

You are old, you are sick, you are poor, and you are forgotten. Most of your life is not before you, it is behind you. Your country's news media consistently report on suicides among young people with little mention that the rate of suicide in your age group is several times higher. You live in an environment full of ageism and are systematically denied opportunities for a meaningful community role. You live, ignored, in a sea of troubles. Your spouse has either died or is in failing health, as you are. It is sad to see what life has come to, and it can lead you to thoughts of ending it all.

The highest rates of suicide in the United States occur among persons older than 70 years—rates that are close to double those among adolescents. Among the elderly, although suicides by men outnumber those by women, the percentage difference is not as great as in younger age groups. This statistic suggests that the forces promoting suicide in the elderly may be similar among women and men. We suspect that a primary cause of these escalating and equalizing suicide rates is not only the natural infirmities of old age but also the disenfranchisement of the elderly from the social fabric of our community. Once their value in the workforce has been exhausted, elderly persons are left to fend for themselves for perhaps two decades or more. Scant social resources are available, and familiar social institutions such as church and family have been stripped of their significance. Some elderly persons make the transition exceedingly well, whereas others struggle mightily to find a meaningful life course.

Although the interventions described in this book can and should be applied to the elderly, several factors make working with older people somewhat clinically complicated. First and foremost is the fact that elderly patients, at least in our times, are not likely to seek treatment from the mental health system. They are far more likely to visit their family physicians, seeking relief from a chronic illness or complaining of a multitude of physical symptoms that mask their emotional distress. For this reason, elderly patients need to be regularly assessed for suicidality by their primary care doctors. Such an assessment is particularly necessary for patients whose health has taken a dramatic turn for the worse, who have recently lost a spouse or life partner, or who have been plunged into social isolation through relocation. In addition to not seeking treatment of suicidality, the elderly do not talk about it much nor do they make as many nonlethal suicide attempts as other age groups. Suicide among the elderly can be an insidious, silent lethality.

An additional concern in working with the elderly patient is that many of the stimuli for suicidality in this group are environmentally driven and realistically represent major challenges to the patient's quality of life. For example, an elderly, nonambulatory patient with chronic lung disease is realistically facing a marked decline in quality of existence. Although these types of difficulties can be successfully handled within the problem-solving model, it takes a clinician who is strongly committed to the inherent value of living to keep the work positive and upbeat in content. Many conventional indicators of quality of life often have been removed from the landscape of the elderly person. Success and satisfaction often revolve around finding spiritual meaning in a life that is in danger of being marked by loneliness, financial worries, and chronic physical illness. Elder abuse may be an increasingly common precipitant of suicidal behavior, particularly when the perpetrator is a family member who is charged to take care of the patient. This type of family turmoil is often so painful for the elderly patient to acknowledge that suicide seems to be the only way of saving face.

It is sometimes difficult to know the role that psychiatric illness, particularly depression, plays in suicidal behavior in an elderly person. Demoralization can be mistaken for signs of clinical depression. Demoralization consists of separate responses to specific environmental losses. The demoralized elderly patient has been let down by society and, to a larger extent, by life. Plans for a happy retirement are suddenly demolished upon the unexpected death of a spouse; dreams of financial security in retirement years give way to living on an inadequate fixed income; and many friends and loved ones die, change residences, or move into nursing homes. These demoralizing events can dash hopes for a productive, relatively worry-free late life. The sadness and loss of interest that result from these events can precipitate suicidality, which can be addressed by a problem-solving approach. Be judicious in using antidepressant medications to treat this age group. Pills work only when the patient takes them as directed, and they never work when taken all at once. Pills do not necessarily cause other people to change, and they rarely cause pensions to increase. Demoralization is caused by tangible problems. Find out about problems, and develop an overall plan to deal with them.

The approach to treatment of an elderly patient involves helping him or her accept the very real changes that have occurred in life related to aging. Living to be 89 and frail with end-stage congestive heart disease is not as much fun as it sounds. On the other hand, just living for living's sake is not really living at all. It is a lifeless outcome produced by the miracles of modern medical technology. Teach the patient that living for something means incorporating losses, physical discomfort, and the like into a new life plan. It also involves building a value-based problem-solving approach, which may include finding a new set of life supports or a plan to restore interest in spiritual or personal growth activities. Rather than allowing your patient to give up and withdraw from life, emphasize opportunities available for meeting new people. If physical disease has eliminated some of your patient's traditional leisure time and recreational activities, make sure the search is on for alternative types of leisure and recreation that will continue to challenge your patient's sense of independence and physical capability. In other words, rather than challenging beliefs about what types of losses have occurred, acknowledge that the losses have occurred and set up treatment so that rebuilding is possible. Finding the spark that makes life a continued challenge and joy is the crux of the therapeutic task for suicidal elderly patients.

Development of a competent social support network is perhaps the most important single factor in treatment. Self-help groups, peer support, and an organized approach by the family's younger generation are most important.

The grown children of the older suicidal person can feel overwhelmed and powerless. Work with them. In particular, help them to find the limits of what they can and cannot do, especially in the context of raising their own families. For example, an elderly woman living alone had a great fear of accident or illness and insisted that her daughter call her every day. The daughter lived in a different city, and although she wanted to help, she came to resent both the demand and the expense. The relationship deteriorated. The mother recognized the effects of her demands, but the fears persisted. Demoralization set in. The answer? Voice mail. Each day, at her expense, the mother would call and leave a message: "Hi, everybody. I'm OK." Mother and daughter agreed that if the mother did not leave a message, the daughter would call and check. Otherwise, they talked on the phone about once a week, a level of contact that was satisfying to both mother and daughter.

Helpful Hints

- Know your medications and their side effects. Remember to watch for dysphoria, agitation, akathisia, and akinesia.
- Avoid polypharmacy when you can.
- Give medications a trial. If a medication is not working, stop it or change it.
- Consult with your fellow practitioner when you are working with the same patient.
- Substance abuse and suicidality cannot be treated as completely separate entities. Individuals who work with one must be able to work with the other.
- Substance abuse in all its forms can produce almost any psychiatric symptom, including suicidality.
- Be persistent in asking about suicidality when you suspect or know of substance abuse.
- Integrate substance abuse in the context of suicidality.
- Include substance abuse in your crisis management plan.
- If a problem behavior occurs in a session (e.g., drunkenness), try to understand it and use the information to the patient's advantage.
- Actively inquire about mood change and suicidal thinking on detoxification units.

- In working with schizophrenic patients, assess suicidality, know your medications, and be very practical in your approach.
- Always assess a suicidal adolescent's family.
- The elderly are the most suicidal age group, and effective treatment must address the real-world challenges associated with aging.

References

American Psychiatric Association: Diagnostic and Statistical Manual of Mental Disorders, 4th Edition, Text Revision. Washington, DC, American Psychiatric Association, 2000

Chiles JA, Miller AL, Crismon ML, et al: The Texas Medication Algorithm Project: development and implementation of the schizophrenia algorithm. Psychiatr Serv 50:69–74, 1999

Healy D: Lines of evidence on the risks of suicide with selective serotonin reuptake inhibitors. Psychother Psychosom 72:71–79, 2003

Tondo L, Hennen J, Baldessarini RJ: Lower suicide risk with long term lithium treatment in major affective illness: a meta-analysis. Acta Psychiatr Scand 104:163–172, 2001

Selected Readings

Allebeck P, Varla A, Kristjansson E, et al: Risk factors for suicide among patients with schizophrenia. Acta Psychiatr Scand 76:414–419, 1987

Bartels SJ, Drake RE, McHugo GJ: Alcohol abuse, depression, and suicidal behavior in schizophrenia. Am J Psychiatry 149:394–395, 1992

Blazer DG, Bachar JR, Manton KG: Suicide in late life: review and commentary. J Am Geriatr Soc 34:519–525, 1986

Chiles, JA, Carlin AS, Benjamin GA I, et al: A physician, a nonmedical psychotherapist, and a patient: the pharmacotherapy-psychotherapy triangle, in Integrating Pharmacotherapy and Psychotherapy. Edited by Beitman BD, Klerman GL. Washington, DC, American Psychiatric Press, 1991, pp 105–118

De Wilde EF, Kienhorst I, Diekstra R, et al: The relationship between adolescent suicidal behavior and life events in childhood and adolescence. Am J Psychiatry 149:45–51, 1992

Hawton K, Fagg J: Deliberate self-poisoning and self-injury in adolescents: a study of characteristics and trends in Oxford, 1976–89. Br J Psychiatry 161:816–823, 1992

Miller ML, Chiles JA, Barnes VE: Suicide attempters within a delinquent population. J Consult Clin Psychol 50:491–498, 1982

Murphy GE, Wetzel RD: Multiple risk factors predict suicide in alcoholism. Arch Gen Psychiatry 49:459–463, 1993

Power AC, Cowen PJ: Fluoxetine and suicidal behaviour: some clinical and theoretical aspects of a controversy. Br J Psychiatry 161:735–741, 1992

Rich CL, Young D, Fowler RC: San Diego Suicide Study; I: young vs old subjects. Arch Gen Psychiatry 43:577–582, 1986

Shear M, Frances A, Weiden P: Suicide associated with akathisia and depot fluphenazine treatment. J Clin Psychopharmacol 3:325–326, 1983

Westermeyer JF, Harrow M, Marengo JT: Risk for suicide in schizophrenia and other psychotic and nonpsychotic disorders. J Nerv Ment Dis 179:259–266, 1991

10

Suicidal Patients in General Health Care

General health care has undergone a rather radical transformation since the early 1990s. We have witnessed a transition from health care functioning in an acute care model primarily oriented toward serving the ill to a model of health care that emphasizes prevention and chronic disease management. The role of the primary care provider has been similarly transformed. In general, patient examinations are shorter and more balanced between acute care, chronic disease management, and preventive health care functions. Primary care providers typically see more patients in a practice day than was the case a decade ago, simply because population health models rely heavily on providing at least basic medical services to most of the community. For many patients, the general practitioner is the first point of contact in the process of accessing services, whether it is health services, mental health services, or addiction treatment services. Like it or not, there is still a tendency in Western civilization to visit the "doctor" to first bring up personal difficulties. Numerous studies have shown that psychosocial issues drive most general health care services. Research findings also have suggested that the last provider seen by a patient before a completed suicide is likely to be a general health practitioner. Even though medical providers lack the specialized training given to mental health providers, their patients do not make that discrimination. At the end of the day, quality health care must involve paying attention not only to the body but also to the mind.

General health care practitioners need to be effective at treating suicidal behavior in their patients for at least three compelling and clear reasons. First, and most important, the Epidemiologic Catchment Area Program study (Narrow et al. 1993) contained a somewhat startling revelation about the role of general practitioners in delivering mental health care in the United States. Specifically, nearly *one-half* of all patients with mental disorders received their mental health care *solely* from a general practitioner. The impact of this fact on medical practice is made even clearer when we realize that various surveys have shown that medical providers spend as much as one-half of their practice time directly managing mental disorders and chemical addictions. Although suicidality is certainly not limited to people with mental disorders, knowledge of suicidal behavior is part and parcel of dealing with this population. Second, the type of mental disorder treated by the general practitioner is important. Studies of the prevalence of mental disorders among medical outpatients have consistently shown that anywhere from 6% to 10% have a condition that meets diagnostic criteria for major depressive disorder, panic disorder, generalized anxiety disorder, or somatization disorder. The Medical Outcomes Study (Wells et al. 1992) showed that mental disorders are generally underrecognized in general health care settings. A common mental disorder in such settings is *depression,* and one of the diagnostic symptoms of depression is *suicidal ideation or behavior.* Third, because of financial or resource limitation, many suicidal medical patients do not have access to mental health care. There are both rural and urban parts of the United States that have poor to nonexistent mental health care resources. There may be few, if any, mental health providers in these areas. Even when referral for mental health care is available and acceptable to a suicidal patient, considerable travel time may be required to attend sessions, and access to the mental health provider may be severely limited. In these situations, if a crisis develops, it is going to be the initial responsibility of the general practitioner to manage it. In sum, in a large number of cases, the patient will receive all treatment in the general health care practitioner's office—the major de facto mental health system in the United States.

The general health care clinic can be a most difficult arena in which to properly address suicidality. There is much going on, decisions must be made quickly, and the database is often incomplete. When a patient is suicidal, the situation is usually emotionally charged, and the push to do something quickly can often seem overwhelming. Suicidal patients do not always fit easily into a setting that relies on evaluation, focused treatment, and long intervals between follow-up visits. To deal with suicidality, health care providers must have a thorough understanding of both their personal and clinical responses to the suicidal patient. If you are a health care provider, we would strongly recommend that you review Chapter 2 ("The Clinician's Emotions, Values, Legal Exposure, and Ethics") to evaluate how your own moral, emotional, and legal concerns may influence how you respond to such patients. As do those of mental health providers, your "hot buttons" can get in the way of doing good work with suicidal patients.

Many general health care practitioners believe that it is very difficult, if not impossible, to conduct anything resembling an effective intervention with the suicidal patient within the confines of a busy schedule with patient visits spaced 15 minutes apart. General practitioners point to the full 50-minute session used by mental health providers and rightly wonder how a 15-minute (or even 5-minute) intervention can be done when trained specialists take up to an hour. *The key difference is the context—the general health care setting is one in which things happen rapidly, and most patients have a certain readiness for this.* The mental health context is oriented toward the process of deliberate and detailed discussions focused on producing change in many aspects of the patient's life. At times, the general health care provider has a distinct advantage over the mental health therapist, notwithstanding the fast pace of primary health care visits. Both practitioner and patient are acclimated to a setting in which action is expected, the instructions are crisp, and adherence is high. This acclimation evolves from the long-term, sometimes lifelong, relationship the primary care provider has with the patient and the fact that the provider is seen as a trusted, friendly physician, not an imposing, inquiry-driven stranger. Despite the strengths of this special kind of leverage, many general practitioners still routinely respond with a not-in-my-office approach and try to refer the suicidal patient to some form of psychiatric treatment. This action is often based on the premise that the patient needs to be discharged from the general health care system and admitted to a mental health care system. It is a premise not always fulfilled. Many times, a gap of days and even weeks occurs between the patient's leaving one system and entering another, if the transfer happens at all. In some clinical settings, as many as three-fourths of the patients referred from general health care never arrive for a mental health appointment. A common referral practice, and one that sometimes seems set up to fail, is to give a patient a phone number with instructions to call for an appointment. The patient may not call. It is one more impersonal task to perform. Your patient may get one (or more) busy signals and become discouraged. Even worse, the patient is faced with a recorded message and runs the risk of getting lost in the infamous voice mail jail. Almost as discouraging is to be told by a harried clinic clerk that no appointments are available for a month or so. In these eventualities, your patient remains in limbo, and you remain in a position of potential liability for a negligence suit in the event of an adverse outcome. Our recommendation is to solidify your transfer relationships with documented confirmation that continuity of care has been accomplished. In addition, develop your procedures for managing the period that is so overlooked and so important—the *in the meantime*. In the remainder of this chapter we discuss those procedures, and we hope the discussion will give you the tools you need for treating these patients within your clinic structure.

Develop Quick, Effective Screens for Suicidality

We discuss assessment of suicidality in Chapter 4 ("Assessment of Suicidal Behavior and Predisposing Factors"). These assessments can be conducted in a variety of settings, take varying amounts of time, and are used to gather various types of information. One essential rule pertains to any assessment procedure: *It is part of treatment.* A reasonable and caring assessment, even a 10-minute one, leaves the patient with the understanding that the problem has been taken seriously and that help is on the way. Assessment in general health care should be proactive regarding suicidal behaviors. All patients should be screened for suicidal thoughts and behavior as part of an initial health care assessment. Questions about suicidality should be a regular part of the screening examination and not be linked to statements about particular psychiatric states such as depression and anxiety, particularly in the increasingly popular structured interview format with its decision-tree method. A common error in screening is to ask about depression and, if the answer is no, to skip questions about suicidal ideation or behavior. Suicidality occurs in many patients who have no diagnosable psychiatric disorder, and some patients who are ultimately found to have a psychiatric disorder initially deny (do not reveal on direct questioning) their symptoms. In other words, *suicidal behavior, ideation, and threats can accompany any psychiatric condition,* and they can be present when no psychiatric condition is diagnosed. Accordingly, these behaviors need to be routinely asked about in a health care assessment.

Appendix D (Suicidal Thinking and Behaviors Questionnaire) is a short form that can be used to assess suicidal history, intensity, causality, and efficacy. This questionnaire provides you with a good basic data set regarding suicidality.

Four Indicators to Look For

Four areas of general psychological functioning pertinent to suicidality can be quickly assessed. All of these areas have some long-term (not short-term) predictive power for suicidal potential and are helpful in developing a treatment plan. The first is the *problem-solving efficacy of suicide* (see Appendix D, item 6). This question is used to assess whether a patient believes committing suicide will solve his or her problems. When a person feels that suicide would definitely be effective in dealing with troubles, his or her potential to use suicidal behavior is increased.

The second indicator is *tolerance of emotional distress.* As we outlined in Chapter 3 ("A Basic Model of Suicidal Behavior"), suicidal patients seem unable to tolerate the emotional distress they are experiencing. If a patient indicates that he or she cannot tolerate the emotional or physical pain that is present, there is a very good chance the patient will at least consider suicidal behavior.

The third indicator is *hopelessness* or the patient's lack of faith that the future will be any better than the present. Hopelessness has been shown to have some predictive value for long-term suicidal behavior, especially among depressed persons and especially in Western cultures. You can use the Beck Hopelessness Scale, an excellent instrument for systematic assessment of this variable, or you can ask directly about the patient's outlook on the future. *Do not equate hopelessness with depression.* Hopelessness can come from a variety of conditions, including a generally reasonable assessment of one's life circumstance and environment.

The fourth indicator to assess is the *strength of the patient's survival and coping-related beliefs*. These beliefs are the positive reasons for staying alive that your patient may use to buffer the impact of suicidal impulses. The lack of strongly held coping beliefs may remove some resistance to going ahead with suicidal behavior. Recent findings have shown that the importance a patient attaches to survival and coping beliefs can be an important predictor of suicide intent. The Reasons for Living Inventory (Appendix C) Survival and Coping Beliefs scale can be used to measure this indicator, or you can simply ask the patient to give you some reasons he or she would use to not commit suicide, were the thought to occur.

The Role of Diagnostic Screening

Because suicidality is associated with an underlying psychiatric disorder in approximately 50% of cases, assessment for these disorders is important. Treatment of a specific disorder is important in its own right, but you should not assume that the suicidal crisis is taken care of because the psychiatric disorder is being treated. Much of the suicidality in persons with a psychiatric disorder occurs despite treatment. In addition, recall that a considerable percentage of suicidal patients do not meet criteria for having *any* psychiatric diagnosis. The assumption that suicidality automatically means the presence of a mental disorder can lead you on a diagnostic wild goose chase (most often depression is the goose). Make sure diagnostic criteria are met before you administer psychoactive medication. It is very difficult to justify prescribing pills that are subsequently used in an overdose when a solid basis for the prescription is not found in the clinical records. Our approach is to advocate for treatment both of the psychiatric disorder and of the suicidality and to view these goals as separate aspects of good management. Table 10–1 contains a series of questions that are useful in screening for psychiatric illness. The answer of yes to any question should lead to further evaluation of that psychiatric condition. You can use this instrument to help you determine whether further consultation may be helpful in diagnosis or treatment.

Table 10–1.   Screening for psychiatric illness that may have co-occurring suicidality

Yes ○   No ○   1.   (**Panic disorder/agoraphobia with panic attack**) Has patient ever had spells like a heart attack when became suddenly frightened, anxious, and had chest pain, tightness, trouble breathing, etc.?

Yes ○   No ○   2.   (**Generalized anxiety disorder**) Has patient ever had a period of 6 months or more when most of time nervous, anxious, with bodily symptoms such as weakness, fatigue, stomach problems, muscle aches, etc.?

Yes ○   No ○   3.   (**Depression**) Has patient ever had a period of 2 weeks or more when felt sad, blue, depressed, loss of interest, loss of energy, hopeless, helpless, worthless, etc.?

Yes ○   No ○   4.   (**Dysthymia**) Has patient ever had periods of depressed days with symptoms not every day for 2 weeks over a 2-year period (sporadic symptoms)?

Yes ○   No ○   5.   (**Posttraumatic stress disorder**) Does patient have a history of traumatic event or experience that has led to reexperiencing the trauma (flashbacks) and/or chronic hypervigilance (easily startled, jumpy)?

Yes ○   No ○   6.   (**Mania/hypomania**) Has patient ever had a period of 1 week or more when so happy, excited, irritable, or "high" that patient got into trouble, or family or friends worried about it, or a physician said that patient was manic?

Yes ○   No ○   Has patient ever had a period of at least several days when irritable, "high," or excited, very energetic, very impulsive or confident, or needed less sleep?

Yes ○   No ○   7.   (**Schizophrenia**) Has patient ever heard voices or seen visions?

Yes ○   No ○   Has patient ever believed people were controlling, spying on, following, or plotting against patient, or reading patient's mind?

Yes ○   No ○   Has patient ever believed patient could actually hear or feel other people's thoughts or that other people could actually hear or feel patient's thoughts or put thoughts into patient's mind?

Yes ○   No ○   8.   (**Alcohol/substance abuse**) Has patient ever had problems from drinking alcohol or taking illicit or prescription drugs?

Yes ○   No ○   Desire to Cut down use?

Yes ○   No ○   Have others been Annoyed at patient's use?

Yes ○   No ○   Guilt about use? ("Paranoid")

Yes ○   No ○   "Eye opener" to avoid withdrawal symptoms?

Yes ○   No ○   Has patient ever used marijuana, LSD, cocaine, or stimulants?

Table 10–1.   Screening for psychiatric illness that may have co-occurring suicidality *(continued)*

	CAGE Alcohol C___ A___ G___ E___
	CAGE Substance C___ A___ G___ E___
Yes ○ No ○ **9.**	**(Borderline personality disorder)** Does patient have history of emotional instability, intense and unstable relationships, periods of emotional numbness or emptiness, impulsive self-defeating behavior, or self-mutilating behavior?

Advanced Age and Poor Health Status Should Trigger a Suicidality Assessment

As a general practitioner, be aware of two conditions in which the assessment of suicidality is particularly important. The first is *age*. Although much has been made in the literature about suicides among the young, especially from adolescence through the middle twenties, the most lethal suicidality group is the elderly. Rates of suicide among persons older than 75 years are more than twice as high as rates in the teenage and young adult population. The second condition, often linked to age, is *general state of health*. Both chronically poor health and recent deterioration in health should immediately set in motion a suicide risk assessment. These factors, especially when combined with a current mental disorder such as depression, present a potentially lethal mixture. Many people who have committed suicide have seen a general physician a short time before their death, and these patients often are of advanced age and in poor health. A particularly worrisome situation occurs when both members of a couple are aged and in very ill health. Although you may not be able to predict or prevent a suicide in these situations, simply asking about the patient's life outlook may trigger a much-needed discussion about end-of-life planning, advance directives, and the patient's general outlook on living.

After Detection, Assign an Urgency Level

After determining that there is some degree of suicidality in your patient, the next question is, How much suicidality is there? As we discuss in Chapter 1 ("Introduction: The Dimensions of Suicidal Behavior"), suicidal behavior has many different forms. The three most common forms you will encounter are suicidal ideation (thinking about suicide), suicidal communication (telling someone one is thinking about suicide), and suicide attempt (trying to kill oneself). Most of the time, you will be working with a person who is thinking about suicide or communicating that message to you or someone else. It is important that you gauge the frequency (how often does it occur?), intensity (how specific and detailed are the thoughts or communications?), and duration (how long do the periods of suicidality last?) of the behavior. In general, as frequency, intensity, and duration increase, the patient's sense of urgency escalates. This information, along with an assessment of the four potential indicators of suicide described earlier (see Develop Quick, Effective Screens for Suicidality), will help you make an assessment of urgency of the situation. That is, will the patient need immediate hospitalization or some other form of intensive clinic-based intervention? Hospitalization certainly has its place in the care of a suicidal individual but can be unnecessary and therefore potentially counterproductive. Sometimes the patient is not committable and will not agree to hospitalization, often because of perceived stigma and sense of loss of control. In Chapter 8 ("Hospitals and Suicidal Behavior") we present a detailed decision-making process that should lead to rational use of this intensive and expensive treatment modality. Experience in primary care suggests that hospitalization is a rare occurrence and one that is reserved for the most extreme suicidal emergencies. What that leaves is a large number of patients with significant suicidality that will have to be managed over time in the health care clinic.

So My Patient Is Suicidal....Now What Do I Do?

We focus on seven basic intervention targets (Table 10–2) that will help you and your patient work through a suicidal crisis. You can follow these guidelines to support your patient until transfer to another system of care is accomplished. When transfer is not possible, these steps will give you a framework for addressing suicidality for a longer term. These interventions flow from the information gleaned from the assessment described earlier in this chapter and are designed to initiate and promote nonsuicidal problem solving in your patient.

Target 1: Validate Emotional Pain

The first step is to validate the patient's sense of emotional pain. In Chapter 5 ("Outpatient Interventions With Suicidal Patients"), we discuss using the

Table 10–2.   Seven intervention targets for the suicidal patient

1.   Validate emotional pain.
2.   Discuss ambivalence and provide encouragement to come down on the side of life.
3.   Create a positive action plan.
4.   Develop a crisis management plan.
5.   Connect the patient to local treatment and support resources.
6.   Provide interim emotional support through follow-up phone calls.
7.   Start treatment for psychiatric disorder if indicated.

three *I*s to frame the pain a person feels during a suicidal period: the pain is inescapable, intolerable, and interminable. Communicating an understanding of the pain and legitimizing it for the patient is critical to defusing suicidal impulses. Many suicidal individuals do not see their emotional pain as legitimate. They see it as a flaw, somehow a product of their own weakness. Validating pain is not the same as agreeing that suicide is the only option. If anything, providers are often so worried about inadvertently increasing a patient's suicidal intent that the overall approach can be unnecessarily brusque, leaving the patient with a feeling of lack of empathy. In the midst of a suicidal crisis, there is a terrible sense of isolation, stigmatization, and shame. It helps your patient to make contact with someone who is nonjudgmental and understands the fear and sense of desperation. Validate the pain and at the same time understand that your patient is having trouble thinking through various approaches and solutions to problems. You need to emphasize that the pain is quite understandable given the circumstances but that the method of dealing with the circumstances is faulty. Remember that your patient is often doing the reverse. He or she is assuming that the pain is not legitimate but that the methods of dealing with it are.

Target 2: Discuss Ambivalence and Provide Encouragement to Come Down on the Side of Life

An assumption all health care workers should make is that every suicidal patient is ambivalent: There is both a desire to live and a desire to die. If your patient were absolutely intent on committing suicide, he or she would do it. Lethal means abound. But this is not the case. Your patient is here in the clinic talking to you. Some degree, some glimmer of ambivalence has brought the patient to your office. In other words, your patient has regretfully and in an uncertain manner come to the conclusion that death is the only way out. This conclusion is probably based on the belief that less extreme solutions have already been tried and have failed. The problem for you to address is that your patient's goals were unrealistic (e.g., to stop feeling bad in the midst of a drawn-out antagonistic divorce), poor solutions were used, or good solutions were not used long enough. It is important to come down unequivocally on the positive and life-sustaining part of the patient's ambivalence and to do this without taking a moralistic stance. Your first task is to give voice to your genuine optimism that problems can be solved and that there is more than one way out. A good way to quantify this ambivalence is to use the Reasons for Living Inventory (Appendix C). You can have your patient fill out the inventory, or you can familiarize yourself with the questions and use several of them in the interview. It is most helpful to find an area or two of ambivalence and point these out. If all else fails, you can use the fact of the patient's presence: "You are here. I take your being here as an indication that you are struggling with this issue. Our job is to take the time to look at that struggle. I know it seems very difficult right now to think through things and produce changes, but part of you wants to do that. Certainly, I want to do that. So let's get started."

Validating emotional pain and discussing ambivalence creates a context in which it is possible to provide healthy encouragement to the patient to stay alive and solve problems. The proper use of this technique has as much to do with your attitude and demeanor as it does with what you say. By truly understanding both your patient's pain and your patient's sense of no way out, you will come across as a caring person who can be trusted. If you do not make this connection, your own uncertainty and ambivalence are liable to shine through. Many individuals in the midst of their distress are quite perceptive, especially to nonverbal clues. Your words, the sense of organization you portray, the ability you have to understand what's going on, and your overall confidence level about this approach being the right one are major factors in reassuring and encouraging your patient.

Target 3: Create a Positive Action Plan

Many health care practitioners are trained to seek a no-suicide contract from the patient as a chief intervention strategy and to consider hospitalization if the patient is unwilling to agree to the contract. *We believe that the no-suicide contract is an ineffective intervention strategy.* We detail criticisms of this approach in Chapter 7 ("Managing Suicidal Emergencies"). The main thing we find objectionable about no-suicide contracts is that they specify what the patient is *not* going to do but fail to specify what the patient *is* going to do. Use of a no-suicide contract seems to suggest that treatment is succeeding as long as the patient is not engaging in suicidal behavior. This approach defeats the very basic assumption that suicidal behavior is a form of problem-solving behavior. There are problems that need to be solved; the patient has to "get in motion" and start solving them.

As an alternative, we use the *positive action plan* (see Chapter 7). It is important to remember that when the patient is engaged in reinforcing behaviors, it is very difficult to stew in a suicidal crisis. The positive action plan can include a coping plan, such as self-care behaviors (take a warm bath each night), regular exercise, relaxation and mindfulness practice, scheduling social contacts, and reengaging in church-related activities. After the short-term suicidal crisis has passed, the positive action plan may also include specific problem-solving objectives. The goal of the short-term positive action plan is to have the patient plan and engage in behaviors that are life enhancing by nature. These behaviors are the antithesis of suicidal behavior. Be careful not to develop too many behavioral assignments; stay within the patient's current functioning level. In addition, at the point of initial crisis, develop action plans that last 1 or 2 days rather than longer periods. At the point of crisis, emphasize very basic coping strategies. This time may not be the best for having your patient solve very complicated and emotion-laden life problems. That step will come as the emotional and cognitive functioning of your patient stabilizes. You or a nurse can follow up on the phone to evaluate how the plan is proceeding. Do not be afraid to select small goals. Remember that the rule for motivating positive behavior is to accumulate small successes.

Target 4: Develop a Crisis Management Plan

The crisis card is one of the more useful tools in the management of suicidality. Your patient may actually have used effective strategies to deal with past crises or can brainstorm with you and come up with new ones. However, when the moment is at hand, the patient cannot remember what was discussed or does not follow through in any sort of stepwise manner—hence, the crisis card. Figure 10–1 presents a sample crisis card. Although this sample contains points that are pertinent to many people, it is most important to tailor this card to the individual. The development of such a card usually takes 3–5 minutes at the end of the office visit. The card should contain no more than five or six points. *If your patient has a history of drug or alcohol problems, one item on the crisis card is going to be an instruction to stop any drug or alcohol use if suicidality reappears outside of your office.* The patient should be encouraged to carry the card, make copies, and tell friends and family of the approach. The copies can be put in convenient places around the house and taped to locations such as the medicine chest and the refrigerator. The moment the pain seems to be increasing, the patient should consult the card and follow the steps listed. More information on the crisis card strategy is contained in Chapter 7 ("Managing Suicidal Emergencies").

Target 5: Link Patient to Social and Community Resources

Linking to social and community resources allows your patient to walk away from the office visit with something tangible: a plan of immediate action. In this phase, the physician acts as a case manager, a critical function discussed in Chapter 7 ("Managing Suicidal Emergencies"). This work is easier if professional community resources are available. Who in your clinic or community can work with this individual? Seek these resources out, and discuss referrals with them. Ideally, you should be able to schedule an appointment for your patient while the patient is in the examination room. Remember, requiring the patient to do the legwork can be difficult and discouraging. The suicidal patient already feels stigmatized and may resist making arrangements for outpatient follow-up. Be as helpful as you can. Get your office personnel on the case to make things work smoothly. Remember that even when a referral is set, the problems continue. For this reason, the use of the telephone to deal with interim support is quite important. You may, however, be in a location without professional help. Be creative. Use family, friends, community centers, church groups, social organizations, and whatever else you and your patient can think of. A strength of resource-poor areas is often that the members of the community have a greater willingness to help than that found in the more chaotic and anonymous world of a larger city.

Target 6: Arrange Telephone Follow-Up

Arrange to initiate at least two supportive phone calls in the time between your evaluation and your next visit or the point at which your patient is

---

Crisis card sample

Do not drink, or, if I am drinking, stop drinking.

Sit down and take 50 deep breaths.

Say to myself 10 times, "No matter how bad things are right now, I am a strong person and I will survive."

Contact one of my friends who has said they will help me, and talk for 5 minutes about our joint interests.

Write down why I became upset and how I dealt with things so that I can discuss this episode with Dr. _____ at our next contact.

Figure 10–1.   Crisis card sample.

scheduled to begin long-term treatment. You, a nurse, or other office personnel should organize the call to keep it brief and focused. Use the format outlined in Table 10–3. These calls are not meant to be therapy sessions. They are meant to display ongoing support and encouragement by following up on points that were made in the initial evaluation. Has your patient had the opportunity to use the crisis card? Have arrangements been made for a specialty mental health appointment? Make your patient understand that you are confident that things will get better if the patient follows through on the plan. Remember that the crisis plan can be modified. If some aspect is not helpful, change it. Encourage your patient to come up with ideas. Develop a sense of partnership in the task. Give a technique a fair trial. If a technique does not work, change it.

Target 7: Initiate Appropriate Medication Treatment

The last intervention is to start medication treatment of any mental disorder you have properly diagnosed. This aspect of care of a suicidal patient can be tricky, and some general health care providers are better trained and more comfortable prescribing medication than are others. Remember that *medica-*

Table 10–3.   Supportive phone call structure

1. State that you are calling as part of the initial plan of treatment.
2. Ask about details of treatment, such as arrangements for future appointments and taking medication as prescribed.
3. Ask about emotional states and use of the crisis card. Has the card been effective? Discuss changes if it has not.
4. End with encouraging statement.

tion in and of itself is not sufficient treatment of suicidality, although it may be highly effective in providing symptom relief. However, do not prescribe medications to your patient if psychiatric symptoms have not been demonstrated. This tactic can backfire. Medications cannot produce change in people, and they do not serve their intended purpose when taken all at once. A good technique is to develop a crisis card before writing a prescription. The pain tolerance and problem-solving techniques embedded in the card directives may be a better and more permanent solution to your patient's difficulties than adding a pill to the mix.

The most common disorder dealt with is depression. However, suicidality is only one symptom of depression and is not sufficient for making the diagnosis. You need to carefully review the other diagnostic symptoms of this disorder before assuming that antidepressant medications are necessary. The most important consideration in prescribing medication for a suicidal depressed patient is the type of drug used and total amount of medication given. Until recently, we would have said that a safe medicine class to use is the selective serotonin reuptake inhibitors (SSRIs), such as fluoxetine, sertraline, and paroxetine. These medications require little or no titration for most patients. The overdose potential is quite small, and these drugs can be prescribed for intervals that match the patient's overall treatment program. However, in the spring of 2003 the U.S. Food and Drug Administration (FDA) issued a warning on the use of paroxetine in the treatment of patients younger than 18 years because of the possibility that the drug can trigger suicidality in vulnerable individuals. This decision was based in large measure on results of a reanalysis of the FDA randomized clinical trial database comparing placebo- with paroxetine-treated patients. There have been anecdotal reports claiming iatrogenic suicidality in some patients treated with SSRIs beginning in the early 1990. We urge you to keep abreast of this issue. Our position for some time has been that no antidepressant medication has been shown effective in reducing suicidal behavior. We are concerned that reanalysis of the FDA databases on new antidepressant medication may move some of these medications from a neutral to a harmful position for some of our suicidal patients. We discuss this issue in Chapter 9 ("Working With Special Populations").

Antianxiety agents, in particular benzodiazepines, may be used for very short periods to allay the acute overarousal associated with suicidal crisis. Beyond the very short term, antianxiety agents are of limited usefulness in treating suicidality. These drugs often produce sedation, a state that is usually *not* conducive to increased autonomy and self-efficacy. Benzodiazepines are effective in the treatment of anxiety *if* you have established that an anxiety disorder is present. These agents can be used to treat insomnia if you are convinced that the short-term treatment of sleeplessness would be helpful, but there are better chemical agents for that type of problem. The dangers of extended use of antianxiety drugs are well known: the development of tolerance and the possible need for increasing doses, dependency, and the sometimes horrendous problem of withdrawal after long-term use. So think about these agents carefully. We have found antianxiety drugs overused in the care of suicidal individuals. The short-term palliative effects of these drugs on highly aroused patients often do not provide sufficient benefit to justify use.

Helpful Hints

- Even in the context of a busy practice, the general health care provider can create an atmosphere in which good things happen for a suicidal patient.
- Use Table 10–1 to set up an assessment of suicidality as part of your screening procedures.
- Train your staff to use telephone follow-up in a brief, focused, and empathetic manner.
- Develop your referral sources. Make your office part of a system that cares for the suicidal patient.

Reference

Wells KB, Burnam MA, Rogers W, et al: The course of depression in adult outpatients. Results from the Medical Outcomes Study. Arch Gen Psychiatry 49:788–794, 1992

Selected Readings

Beck A, Steer RA, Kovacs M, et al: Hopelessness and eventual suicide: a 10 year prospective study of patients hospitalized with suicidal ideation. Am J Psychiatry 142:559–563, 1985

Beck A, Weissman A, Lester D, et al: The measurement of pessimism: the Hopelessness Scale. J Consult Clin Psychol 42:861–865, 1974

Chiles JA, Carlin AS, Benjamin GAH, et al: A physician, a nonmedical psychotherapist, and a patient: the pharmacotherapy-psychotherapy triangle, in Integrating Pharmacotherapy and Psychotherapy. Edited by Beitman BD, Klerman GL. Washington, DC, American Psychiatric Press, 1991, pp 105–118

Hawton K, Catalan J: Attempted Suicide: A Practical Guide to its Nature and Management, 2nd Edition. New York, Oxford University Press, 1987

Michel K, Valach L: Suicide prevention: spreading the gospel to general practitioners. Br J Psychiatry 160:757–760, 1992

Murphy GE: The physician's role in suicide prevention, in Suicide. Edited by Roy A. Baltimore, MD, Williams & Wilkins, 1986, pp 171–179

Narrow WE, Regier DA, Rae DS, et al: Use of services by persons with mental health and addictive disorders: findings from the National Institute of Mental Health Epidemiologic Catchment Area Program. Arch Gen Psychiatry 50:95–107, 1993

Von Korff M, Shapiro S, Burke S, et al: Anxiety and depression in a primary care clinic. Arch Gen Psychiatry 44:152–156, 1987

Wells K, Hays R, Burnam M, et al: Detection of depressive disorder for patients receiving pre-paid or fee for service care. JAMA 262:3293–3302, 1988

11

Understanding and Providing Care to the Survivors of Suicide

Patricia J. Robinson, Ph.D.

The people in the life of a person who has committed suicide who were close to him or her are the survivors of suicide. Unfortunately, understanding and treating survivors of suicide is not receiving adequate attention in empirical investigations. Available results of studies suggest that group treatment of survivors results in a lowering of psychosomatic symptoms. In addition, survivors differ from other bereaved individuals in their experience of bereavement processes and in their vulnerability to mental health symptoms. Little is known about the process factors in the demise or healing of survivors. I attempt to bridge this gap by offering a theoretical framework for exploring the functioning and healing of the growing number of survivors.

Although survivors of suicide have a great deal in common with victims of other losses, their bereavement may be prolonged and more complex (Allen et al. 1993–1994; Brent et al. 1994). On a psychiatric symptom checklist, survivors endorsed more symptoms overall than did psychiatric outpatients.

Specifically, survivors endorsed more somatization, obsessive-compulsive, depression, anxiety, and paranoid ideation symptoms (Grad 1996a). At least one-half reported clinically significant symptoms of depression, and adults who lost a child to suicide were even more likely to be devastated by depression. Child survivors are also more at risk of psychiatric symptoms and impaired functioning than are adults (Calhoun and Allen 1992–1993; Saarinen et al. 1999; Seguin et al. 1995; Silverman 1994–1995). Among children 5–14 years of age who had experienced the suicidal death of a relative within the past year, 25% reported clinically significant symptoms of depression, 40% reported moderate to severe symptoms of posttraumatic stress disorder, and more than 30% reported suicidal ideation (Pfeffer et al. 1997). As might be expected, surviving children experience more problems when their parents are more symptomatic (Pfeffer et al. 1997).

Unfortunately, few survivors seek care for their suffering, and their functioning stagnates or declines over time (Knieper 1999; Saarinen et al. 1999). In part, this reluctance relates to the survivors' experience of confusion and shame (Seguin et al. 1995). Many withdraw from social contacts and may fail to perceive efforts of support (Reed 1993; Reed and Greenwald 1991; Wagner and Calhoun 1991–1992). On the other hand, research findings suggest that support offered to suicide survivors may be significantly less than that offered to other bereaved individuals (Farberow et al. 1992a). When survivors seek care, they may go to a medical rather than a behavioral health care setting and present with medical complaints. In the case of children and youth, the struggle is most likely to be acted out in school, where many students experience social and academic failure. Postvention programs in schools are usually brief and intensive in nature, and the lack of follow-up may leave many youths without a bridge to connect them to ongoing behavioral health care. Women survivors are more likely to perceive a need for behavioral health care than are men (Grad 1996b). Therefore, men may be even more at risk. The high risk is particularly true of men who engage in readily available and powerful methods of psychological avoidance, such as abuse of alcohol and illegal drugs.

Several factors appear to influence the impact of suicide on a survivor. The closeness of the relationship rather than kinship per se is predictive of the intensity and length of postsuicide struggle and suffering. The overall vulnerability of the individual plays a significant role, and social support is potentially a strong buffer (Farberow et al. 1992b). Unfortunately, almost one-third of the participants in a survivor's support group reported having no one or only one person in their lives whom they counted on to understand how they felt (Gaffney et al. 1992). Survivors with lower self-esteem are less likely than persons with high self-esteem to avail themselves of social support, including participation in religious activities. Survivors with lower self-esteem also are more likely to develop more distant relationships with their families.

Survivors appear to receive less support and more negative evaluations than other bereaved individuals (Moore 1995). Blame and responsibility were more prevalent in the responses of college students who witnessed a film of a bereaved woman if told that the loss was due to suicide rather than to an accidental or natural cause (Allen et al. 1993–1994). Undergraduates are particularly negative toward survivors who are stepparents—as opposed to biological parents—of a suicide victim (Calhoun and Allen 1992–1993). As a group, survivors tend to rate themselves as receiving less support than their supporters see themselves as giving and report feeling pressured to recover. Many survivors become caught in a negative feedback of not recognizing support when it is offered, not reinforcing supporters, and then withdrawing further from others in anticipation of a lack of support. It is in this context that the prevailing view of the survivor—only another survivor of suicide can understand—makes sense.

Trauma is probably a huge factor in survivor response to the completed suicide (Orcutt 2002). The level of trauma resulting from loss of a loved one to suicide is directly related to the level of attachment and the directness of exposure to the suicide (Elliott 1997). Being witness to a loved child's suicide is probably the most traumatic exposure. In addition, trauma history before the suicide is an important predictor of survivor response. Survivors of suicide as a group, along with suicide victims, have histories replete with more loss experiences and early separations from parents, in comparison with bereaved individuals losing loved ones to accidental death (Seguin et al. 1995). Research findings by J.M.G. Williams (2003) at Oxford University in the United Kingdom suggest that victims of traumatic experiences—particularly those that occurred in early childhood—may develop information-processing deficits that predispose them to use of defective problem-solving strategies, delayed rates of acquiring new information, and, in many cases, chronic, intermittent depression. Individuals experiencing early trauma are more likely to have overly general responses to emotionally laden stimuli and to lack the ability to easily integrate current experiences at verbal and emotional levels. For these individuals, a loss to suicide may be particularly devastating.

In a large self-report survey of victims' next of kin, suicide survivors reported less emotional distress and shock but greater feelings of guilt, shame, and rejection than did survivors of accidental death (Reed and Greenwald 1991). One way of interpreting this finding is to see the guilt, shame, and rejection as verbal experiences that occur for the individual devoid of integration with emotional experience. Without the emotional integration, the individual does not make progress in experiencing and moving through the loss and trauma experience and remains highly vulnerable to grief-anxiety-depression triggers that occur in the natural environment and promote avoidance and withdrawal. Survivors often have difficulties remembering details about the suicide. When questioned, they respond with vague and overly general words and phrases—"Oh, yeah, he passed on a while back. I don't remember much about it." Survey data also suggest that survivors report higher levels of delayed recall of traumatizing events than survivors of many other traumas and in this way are similar to combat veterans and sexual abuse survivors (Elliott 1997).

I hope to help you better understand the survivor and to plan ways of improving recognition and treatment efforts. With a better understanding of the clinical characteristics of survivors, you will be more able to conceptualize opportunities for improving detection and treatment in community and clinical settings. I suggest practical issues related to intervening with survivors and present a three-stage clinical model for treating survivors. Using this model, I suggest a session-by-session guide for group treatment of survivors. I conclude with suggestions for adapting the three-stage model to the primary care setting, in which there are many opportunities for identifying and treating survivors.

Clinical Characteristics of Survivors of Suicide

Although survivors of suicide are individuals and present with a range of problems, eight symptoms tend to be present to some extent in most survivors when they present to a medical or clinical setting. Presentation for treatment is usually triggered by some new stress that exhausts a survivor's coping resources, or someone in his or her life suggests the need for professional treatment. Often the trigger is a problem in role functioning, such as school, job, or relationship problems. The most vulnerable survivors are those with little social support and histories of early loss and trauma. Individuals in this most vulnerable group invariably have histories of intermittent depression, and many have chronic anxiety. However, most have received no treatment other than use of antidepressant medications for brief periods. Understanding the clinical presentation of survivors facilitates better detection. Therefore I integrate suggestions for detection with this discussion of clinical manifestations. Table 11–1 is a summary of the eight symptoms of what might be called survivors of suicide syndrome, along with suggestions for detection.

Table 11–1.   Survivors of suicide syndrome: symptoms and detection strategies

Characteristic or symptom	Detection strategy
1. Often leads highly functional life "on the surface"	1. Primary care and school interview strategies that include discussion of value-based directions in life
2. Avoids the experience of intimacy	2. Focus on value-based directions specific to relationships
3. Complains of lack of motivation or underachievement of life goals	3. Primary care and school interventions that support reactivation of dreams
4. Has vague and diffuse mood complaints (i.e., dysthymia, apprehension)	4. Primary care screening for depression
5. Has inexplicable absence of pleasure, sense of participation	5. Assessment of health-related quality of life
6. Often does not mention the suicide unless asked	6. Inclusion of trauma screening questions with select patients and students
7. Often has memory gaps and avoidance sequences related to the suicide trajectory	7. Inclusion of questions about early trauma
8. Primarily uses idealization and rationalization	8. Collaboration between primary care or school providers and behavioral health providers for integrated treatment

1. *Survivors of suicide often lead very functional lives "on the surface."* They of-
    ten live with other family members and participate in the workforce. I
    have seen several women widowed by a suicide who were relatively strong
    in their role of mother while working full-time jobs. However, they re-
    ported an ongoing pervasive sense of disappointment with life and fal-
    tered with formation of new relationships. Many male survivors are often
    gainfully employed, and many work in leadership roles, in which they are
    respected by fellow workers. Some survivors find the ongoing stress of be-
    ing an unaided survivor and the social demands of jobs held before the
    suicide too taxing and locate alternative positions that are less demanding
    and rewarding. Early in my work with survivors, I met a man who had
    owned his own construction company and sold out in an effort to lower
    his stress level. He began a small parking lot operation but continued to
    suffer from insomnia, nightmares, and chronic worry. Unfortunately, sur-
    vivors are likely to have few friends and few meaningful leisure activities.
    Survivors usually struggle in their intimate relationships, and their resil-
    iency to stress is limited. Even a mild interpersonal stressor, such as a
    child's emergence into adolescence, can trigger a period of dysfunction for
    a parent who has lost a partner to suicide. The facade of adequate func-
    tioning may crumble easily into a chaos of interpersonal suffering.

    Detection: Primary care and school interview strategies that include
    discussion of value-based directions in life may improve identification of
    survivors. Because survivors rarely reveal their loss to suicide up front, dis-
    cussions about how much they like their lives constitute an acceptable ap-
    proach to going beyond the appearance of normality and into the despair
    that is often just below the surface. One question that I often ask is,
    "Would you continue doing what you are doing in your life if no one were
    looking?" Primary care physicians and school counselors are in prime po-
    sitions for initiating these interactions and for linking the survivor to
    other resources.

2. *Survivors of suicide often avoid the experience of intimacy.* Survivors may not
    avail themselves of traditional interpersonal sources for bereavement sup-
    port. They anticipate that they "just wouldn't fit" into a bereavement
    group offered at the funeral home or that their religious leader "wouldn't
    want to hear" about their problems. They may talk less within their fam-
    ilies and avoid conflict more. Although the survivor often sees this shut-

ting-down strategy as a temporary one, it can easily become a new way of living. In some cases, survivors lock in on quieting their emotional turmoil by avoiding any emotional expression and by tenacious tiptoeing around addressing problems involving conflict. In the survivor family, communication may be indirect and somewhat forced. Survivors are often careful about forming new relationships. They often do not want to reveal the story of their loss, because they fear negative judgment, and they seek to avoid taking risks that could lead to further interpersonal loss.

Detection: School counselors and primary care providers, along with behavioral health providers, may boost detection of survivors by asking questions about a student's, patient's, or client's sense of being on track in his or her relationships. In an effort to facilitate these discussions, I often ask one or more of the following questions: Remember a time when you felt very close to your mother (or father, brother, or another person). What were you doing? When you were younger and you thought about being a good friend, what did you think that would involve? When you were younger and you thought about being married, what was your dream of what it would be like? Think for a moment about your favorite romantic movie or television show, and tell me what you like most about the way the two lovers interact.

3. *Survivors of suicide often complain of lack of motivation or of underachievement of life goals.* Survivors readily talk about having not reached their potential and about how they have perhaps let others down. Dysthymia is common among survivors. Interestingly, they often do not cry or show emotion as they present this complaint. Even while complaining of underachievement, survivors may state a goal of just maintaining the status quo. The choice of words is often vague, and the counselor, physician, or behavioral health provider may have difficulty following survivors' reasoning because the stories sound reasonable on the surface and their emotional expression tends to be subdued.

Detection: Survivors need help to become more specific and more focused on what really matters in life. Their avoidance of such discussions is not related to a lack of values or a lack of caring. They simply fear feeling their feelings. I often use a brief exercise to facilitate discussion of values and "response ability" (see Chapter 6, "The Repetitiously Suicidal Patient"). Survivors often cling to very high values but do not connect them to the choices they make on a daily basis. This approach helps the survivor to focus more on present values and choices than on the regretted, painful past and the anticipated future of failure. The exercise in Figure 11–1 is from my book *Living Life Well: New Strategies for Hard Times* (Robinson 1996).

When using the exercise, the teacher, physician, or clinician needs to encourage survivors to develop a clear picture of what living their values would look like in each of the seven areas. I often ask the survivor to "dream" about possible activities that "bring a smile" or a sense of pride. It is important that the survivor, rather than the clinician, create the picture of what living a value in a particular area looks like. For example, a survivor described the following picture of what living her values in talking with others looked like: "We would be looking each other in the eyes a lot, feeling at ease, speaking honestly, and we wouldn't be rushing or hiding anything." With this picture in mind, the clinician can start to explore the psychological barriers that the survivor experiences when starting to move toward this valued way of relating to another human being.

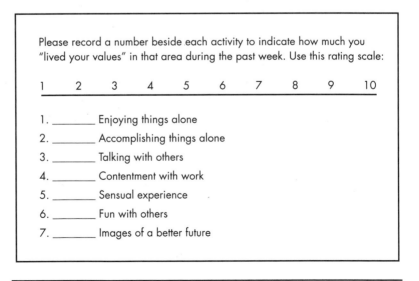

Please record a number beside each activity to indicate how much you "lived your values" in that area during the past week. Use this rating scale:

1   2   3   4   5   6   7   8   9   10

1. _____ Enjoying things alone
2. _____ Accomplishing things alone
3. _____ Talking with others
4. _____ Contentment with work
5. _____ Sensual experience
6. _____ Fun with others
7. _____ Images of a better future

Figure 11–1.   Living Your Values exercise.

4. *Survivors often present with vague and diffuse mood complaints (i.e., dysthymia and apprehension).* In accordance with their sense of underachievement, survivors feel dissatisfied with their lives. They often criticize themselves for feeling dissatisfied, and they struggle with seeking care. Unlike patients with major depression, fewer than one-fourth of survivors seek care from anyone. When they do ask for help, survivors of suicide often present to the medical setting. Given their tendency to look like they are doing okay and to understate their suffering, survivors may go unrecognized until their symptoms of depression are severe and require intensive treatment. A substantial number of survivors also develop generalized anxiety. They worry incessantly about any number of external and internal events, and some develop a pattern of hypervigilance to somatic symptoms. These survivors go to medical settings to report their distress about health problems. The physician understandably explores these symptoms and may not even consider a line of inquiry concerning depression, anxiety, or traumatic loss until after considerable medical workup of the presenting medical complaint.

Detection: Several brief depression questionnaires developed for the primary care setting are available in the public sector for no cost. For example, the Patient Health Questionnaire Nine-Symptom Checklist (PHQ-9; Kroenke et al. 2001) is available online (http://www.american-geriatrics.org/education/dep_tool_05.pdf) and can be administered by a trained nursing assistant as a screening tool in 1 minute and as a depression symptom severity measure in 4 minutes. I often recommend that primary care providers use this questionnaire when a patient's symptoms are not consistent with a disease with an organic basis. In addition, I recommend that providers ask additional questions concerning worry (e.g., Are you a worrier? Do you have trouble controlling your worry, such that you worry a lot—even about small, unimportant things?). When a physician has information about depression and worry, he or she can target these concerns in planning with the survivor.

5. *Survivors often present with an inexplicable absence of pleasure and sense of not participating fully in life.* Survivors use various terms to describe this troubling sense of separation from life. One man who had lost a son to suicide described his experience as having a mud-stained cheesecloth fall over his body, such that his perception of color in life was dulled and his

movements in daily life were less demonstrable and less noticed by others. In a session with me, the man planned to go to a park to look at the plants there, because he had once enjoyed gardening. When he arrived at the park, the man was overcome by sadness when he saw a father and son playing on the playground. He sat on a bench and stared at the dirt below his feet until he "gained control" and walked home. Like my patient, most survivors struggle with lifting the veil of separation because they misunderstand the nature of emotional and cognitive experience and they underestimate their ability to continue to act with intention in the presence of unwanted emotional experience. The legacy of suicide often includes the fusion of intense feeling with the ultimate loss of control—the death of a loved one.

Detection: For the most part, the goal of treatment of survivors is that of improving health-related quality of life. Therefore measures of quality of life are useful for detection as well as for assessing treatment response. As survivors learn to participate more fully in life, their vitality and the day-to-day quality of their lives improve. I use the Duke Health Profile (Parkerson 1996) often in my practice, because I can score it in less than 2 minutes and have scaled scores on physical health, mental health, social health, and perceived health before starting a session with a patient. I usually share these results with patients and explain my reasoning behind ongoing evaluation of functional outcomes associated with treatment.

6. *Survivors often do not mention the suicide unless asked specifically.* Because they are most likely to present to medical rather than behavioral health settings, survivors are not likely to mention the loss to suicide, and they are often not screened by providers concerning a history of traumatic experiences. Even when a survivor does mention the loss to suicide in the primary care setting, the provider may be at a loss as to how to respond in a meaningful way in the context of a 10-minute visit planned to explore a medical complaint. Survivors also may have ambivalent feelings toward medical and behavioral health providers as a result of the quality of care they perceive their loved one received before the completed suicide. If contact with providers of care was negative in regard to the suicide, the survivor may avoid talk of the suicide with providers in an effort to avoid being overcome by sad and angry feelings. Survivors may also fail to mention the loss to suicide as a primary complaint when presenting to a men-

tal health setting. They often focus on unwanted symptoms (i.e., sadness, nervousness, worry, and insomnia) and may not connect these symptoms to the traumatic loss, because the loss often has occurred years before the survivor's presentation for treatment.

Detection: Several brief trauma questionnaires are available, and some of these questionnaires are designed to allow very rapid screening. An example is the Traumatic Life Events Questionnaire (Kubany et al. 2000), which contains 21 items. Although I do not use the entire questionnaire on a routine basis, I often use the following question from it: "Have you experienced the sudden death and unexpected loss of a close friend or loved one?" As with depression and worry, a trained nursing assistant can screen for trauma. When a primary care provider has this information at the beginning of a 10-minute visit, he or she is much more able to have a therapeutic discussion with a survivor, including possible referral to a behavioral health provider. Survivors are most likely to agree to referral to a behavioral health provider and to start treatment if such is available in the primary care setting in an integrated model of care. The primary care behavioral health model (Strosahl 1997) helps to enhance access to behavioral health care and to reduce the stigmatization that often functions as a barrier to treatment of survivors.

7. *Survivors often have memory gaps and avoidance sequences related to the suicide trajectory.* Once a survivor identifies the history of loss to suicide to a medical or behavioral health provider, the caregiver needs to ask questions about the loss. Unfortunately, providers may hesitate in an effort to show respect for the survivor's privacy. Do not hesitate. Ask questions and listen for gaps in the story. Survivors often show confusion about specifics. They may not be sure of the month or day of the suicide, let alone the chronology of the events in the week before the suicide. The more vague the story, the more critical it is for the survivor to challenge it and work to form a story based on more facts.

Detection: A history of early trauma may predispose an individual to information-processing deficits. Clinicians may detect the symptoms of such a deficit by simply asking the survivor to relate a memory of a specific time when he or she was really happy at age 10 (or 12 or 5). Survivors without a history of early trauma often respond with a specific memory— "I tasted hot fudge for the first time. My dad took me to an ice cream store near my grandmother's house." Survivors with a history of early trauma are more likely to give an incomplete and overly general response—"mmmm, yeah, ice cream." With prompts from the clinician, a survivor with early trauma will be able to reconstruct a more specific memory.

8. *Survivors rely primarily on idealization and rationalization in describing the suicide victim and his or her choice to commit suicide.* "He was a good person—his life was just too hard." "I guess he did the best he could." "She didn't really want to hurt anyone." Survivors may offer these as explanations for the suicide victim's choice to commit suicide. These stories often excuse suicide victims and may even make them into heroes. Unfortunately, survivors may distort their lives to support the distorted story.

Detection: Collaboration between primary care providers, school providers, and behavioral health care providers (working in crisis clinics, mental health clinics, and primary care) is critical for optimal detection and treatment of survivors. This collaboration is most likely to happen immediately after a suicide involving a high-profile victim (e.g., a student at a high school, a schoolteacher, or the vice-president of a company). The American Association of Suicidology offers a model for postvention and survivor support services that is designed for easy implementation in any community with support from members of the association. Unfortunately, postvention programs may not be offered to survivors who lose a loved one in the context of a less public setting. I am treating a 12-year-old child who is failing in school and experiencing many problems in his relationship with his mother. When the patient was 8 years of age, he hid inside the house while his father, who was in the front yard, shot himself. This child and others in his family had received no treatment concerning the suicide until 4 years after the fact. Postvention programs are typically brief. Evaluative information on postvention programs in schools suggests that some adolescents may shift back to more romanticized views of suicide several months after completing a postvention program (Callahan 1996). Postvention programs need to incorporate systematic methods for providing follow-up in order to identify survivors who warrant more extensive treatment. All potential providers of care, including police and emergency department staff members, need ongoing training to support optimal detection immediately after—as well as many years after—a suicide.

Practical Issues in Intervening With Survivors of Suicide

For every suicide, there are probably four survivors in need of treatment, and only one in four makes an effort to obtain treatment. In some countries, the suicide rate is increasing. For example, the rate of suicide in the Flemish region of Belgium increased from 15.5 per 100,000 persons in 1991 to 18.9 per 100,000 in 1999. In most communities, the rate of providing support services to survivors is not matched to the number of survivors in need of such services. This gap between need and availability is likely to grow larger during periods of economic stress and war. Only with attention to the details of creating a safety net for the large group of survivors can we hope to intervene meaningfully at a societal level.

A community is most likely to succeed if it obtains funding, public or corporate, to form a representative group charged with creating a network to support survivors of suicide. The membership needs to include representatives from the treatment community (e.g., leaders of survivor groups, crisis care centers, health centers, and schools). Their work needs to support community awareness, use of postvention programs, ongoing training of providers in numerous settings, and promotion of referrals to existing survivor groups. In the United States, November 16 is Suicide Survivors Day. On this day, communities need to facilitate a meeting in which survivors, caregivers, and policy makers can listen to and learn from one other. Local community committees may also develop Web sites that attract survivors and provide information about being a survivor and about local support resources. In addition, the committee needs to include a researcher who can evaluate programs promoted by the committee and provide input for continuing improvement efforts.

A Three-Stage Model for Intervening With Survivors of Suicide

Because psychological avoidance figures prominently in the clinical presentation of the survivor, I rely heavily on acceptance and commitment therapy (ACT) as a theoretical model for conceptualizing treatment (Hayes et al. 1999). The ACT model derives from radical behaviorism and places emphasis on contextual variables in understanding and creating behavior change. The model suggests a distinction between public events (directly observable behaviors) and private events (thoughts, feelings, and sensations). The model also suggests that all behavior, including that of survivors and their providers of support—professional or otherwise—occurs in a complex context influenced by specific variables. Some of these variables can be manipulated or directly changed, whereas others cannot. Context variables that can be manipulated include survivor awareness of survivor programs, survivor attendance at survivor programs or alternative methods of treatment, provider screening that promotes detection, and provider use of effective interventions. Context variables that cannot be directly manipulated include the personal histories and current private events of survivors and providers. These private events are important for providers of care, because their own histories of traumatic loss may hinder their efforts to help survivors. Most providers who have lost a patient to suicide benefit from professional assistance. It is the private events of the survivor that are the focus of attention in the recommended three-stage model.

ACT offers providers a variety of strategies to use with survivors who rely excessively on strategies promoting avoidance of unwanted private events, because these strategies invariably interfere with survivors' organization of daily behaviors, such that choices reflect dearly held values. ACT strategies aim to help survivors reexperience their stories about the suicide, which is in essence a private event, with increased awareness, full emotional experience, and compassion for self. Reexperiencing the story is critical for survivors for two reasons (see Stroebe et al. 2002). First, survivors are unlikely to reevaluate the original story and its impact on their lives without expressed support for the reevaluation. Second, survivors of suicide are likely to receive less compassion from others than are other bereaved individuals and therefore need to generate more of their own compassion for self. ACT strategies include those related to enhancing motivation for change and skills for acceptance of unwanted private experiences, those related to defusing language and perceiving the self as context rather than content, and those related to clarifying values and implementing committed action plans. Table 11–2 summarizes the three-stage model for intervening with survivors. The order of the stages is somewhat arbitrary, in that bits of each stage are often present in most contacts with survivors.

Table 11–2.   Survivors of suicide: a three-stage clinical model

Survivor's work	Theoretical concept	Clinical strategy
I. Awareness of a story and acceptance of the impact of the story		
Identify story about the suicide	Awareness of private events	Who, what, when, how, why, and therefore
		Identify unwanted feelings
		Shovel and hole metaphor
Evaluate benefit-to-cost ratio of the story	Workability of party line	Have patient talk about impact of story on his or her life roles and choices
Reexposure to the traumatic loss through the story	Control as the problem	Educate patient about the private events rule, feeling feelings
		Identify facts of convenience, gaps in knowledge, and black-and-white caricatures
II. Reforming the story and creating more behavioral flexibility		
Re-creation of the story involving full recognition of memories and feelings, data collection to fill in gaps	Defusing language	Have patient write or tell the new story from expanded perspective
		Milk–milk–milk–milk
		Mind: crown of diamonds and of thorns
Having the new story while experimenting with new behaviors	Self as context	Chessboard metaphor
		Passengers on the bus metaphor

Table 11–2. Survivors of suicide: a three-stage clinical model (*continued*)

Survivor's work	Theoretical concept	Clinical strategy
III. Applying the new story to the world		
Moving forward with the new story; using identified gifts as strengths	Valuing	Path up a mountain metaphor Riding a bike metaphor
Initiating greater intimacy and vulnerability	Acting	Developing and implementing life-changing behavior plans

Stage 1: Awareness of a Story and Acceptance of the Impact of the Story

Survivors often do not have a great deal of awareness about their stories concerning the suicide or its impact on life roles. For this reason, perhaps, the top three goals of participation for survivors in a survivors of suicide group program are 1) get the suicide in perspective, 2) deal with family problems caused by the suicide, and 3) feel better about myself. Almost three-fourths of participants describe their main goal as gaining perspective on the suicide. Given the devastating nature of loss by suicide, the survivor usually constructs a rather haphazard story that provides some explanation very soon after the victim's death. This story often is incomplete and distorted and reflects most the need for the survivor to separate from the inexplicable choice the victim made—a choice that disregarded the importance of survivors' feelings and needs. The survivor senses that the perspective is incomplete and wants to talk it out. However, many survivors experience guilt, anticipate blame, and accept the first story without reevaluating it and without examining the impact on the survivor's way of life.

The first story is often incomplete and vague. The following story of Mr. and Mrs. G serves as an example:

Mr. and Mrs. G were middle-aged parents whose only son committed suicide as an adult living in another state. Paul, the son, was an attorney who became despondent over a work problem and shot himself while in his car in a park in a city an approximately 30-minute drive from where he lived with his wife and two young children. Mr. G came to the mental health clinic for treatment of depression. Mr. G also was an attorney and was experiencing work problems and insomnia; his wife had suggested that he come for treatment. The intake worker discovered that Mr. G was a survivor, and Mr. G was offered an opportunity to participate in the survivor of suicide group program. Mr. G agreed and, at the group prescreening, asked whether his wife might participate with him. When asked to relate their who, what, when, how, why, and therefore story to the group, Mr. and Mrs. G's responses included the following:

Who: Our son [Mrs. G]. Our only son [Mr. G].
What: Died, yes died [both].
When: Not sure, a while back [Mrs. G]. A few years ago [Mr. G].
How: Gunshot [both].

Why: Maybe it was an accident [Mrs. G]. Maybe he was having marital problems—and he took the rap for something at work that he didn't do [Mr. G].

Therefore: I don't know how to relate to his wife and his children, so we don't see them very much [Mrs. G]. I have no son, and I don't know what I did wrong [Mr. G].

Upon further questioning by the therapists and the group members, more details emerged. When asked what feelings were most difficult for them, Mr. and Mrs. G responded as follows:

Therapist: And how do you feel when you think that you can't be a grandmother any more?

Wife: Sick, just sick. I just want to go home and lie down and read and forget it. I've gained 25 pounds since it happened, and I don't seem to have the control I used to [tears].

Husband: Guilt.

Therapist: Tell me more about the feeling of guilt.

Husband: I guess scared—like maybe I forgot to do something really important when Paul was little. I forgot to tell him something that he needed when he got in trouble at work.

Therapist: Do you have an idea what that might have been? If you had another chance, what would you say to him?

Husband: I don't know. I told him everything I knew I think. I guess I wished he had known that his suffering would have passed and that way he would have been able to get through it without shooting himself [tears].

Therapist: And right now, when you are suffering with his loss, you know that suffering comes and goes—that it is a part of life as much as joy?

The impact on survivors' lives often becomes apparent as they listen to the story and begin to experience avoided feelings with the benefit of one or more witnesses.

I use a metaphor to help survivors gain greater appreciation of the difficulty of the struggle they are experiencing. The ACT metaphor of a shovel and hole involves asking the survivor to imagine being blindfolded and led onto a field to explore. Unknown to the survivor, there are holes in various places on the field—some small and some large. The survivor begins to walk around and fall in holes. At one point, he hits a hole that is so deep he has trouble climbing out. It's at this point that the survivor notices that he is holding something. It's a bag, and when he opens it, the survivor finds a shovel inside. A shovel is made for digging, so the survivor digs and the hole becomes deeper. The situation is much the same after suicide. Getting rid of guilt, blame, fear, and lack of control by avoiding them does not work. However, given a shovel, most people shovel until they learn to put the shovel down and simply be...in the hole.

I also educate survivors about the rule concerning private events, because they often do not understand it or apply it. In the world of external events, control is a vital strategy. If you don't like cold, build a fire. If you are thirsty, drink water. If someone threatens you, move away from him or her. However, this rule does not apply to internal events, such as thoughts and feelings. I invite survivors to try for a moment not to think of a red Volkswagen. Then I ask them to try not to think of the suicide victim. Most cannot do it for more than 5 minutes, and those who succeed for the 5 minutes then experience a rebound effect whereby they think of the avoided image or thought five times in every 5 minutes.

In addition to eliciting the original story, I encourage survivors to challenge their stories. I ask survivors to question possible facts of convenience. I push for them to remember quotations and, in some cases, to contact others for more information. Stories often have really good and really bad people in them, suggesting the use of caricatures. This tendency is understandable, given the survivor's effort to develop a tight story while being emotionally devastated by the sudden, inexplicable death. In adolescent stories of loss, the victim is usually seen as having been abandoned or abused by an all-bad type of person. It is important to help survivors challenge these overgeneralizations, so that they can develop more cognitive flexibility and create a more accurate story that supports a more vital life.

Stage 2: Reforming the Story and Creating More Behavioral Flexibility

In stage 2, the survivor may benefit from writing the reformed story with full recognition of memories and feelings. This stage is often when gaps in information become obvious, and the survivor is faced with making a choice about how to fill in the gap. I often encourage survivors to look at the options and to evaluate the viability of each option in terms of how it works to support their lives. For example, I worked with a single mother, Ms. P, in her efforts to develop a version of her story for her 9-year-old daughter:

> Ms. P was separated from her husband at the time of his suicide, and she had initiated the separation. The husband had experienced recurrent depression and had abused alcohol throughout the marriage. One evening, he overdosed on a combination of prescription drugs and alcohol. Ms. P struggled with formulating a way to explain to her daughter why the girl's father had committed suicide. Ms. P considered the following options and evaluated the impact of each on her life and possibly on her daughter's life:
>
> > Option 1: He lacked the courage to seek treatment and to resolve his problems with depression, alcohol, and relationships. *Impact:* The daughter may see herself as lacking in courage, because she is her father's daughter, and she may blame her mother in an effort to lessen the believability of the courage explanation (i.e., my mother made my dad feel uncourageous because she abandoned him).
> >
> > Option 2: He mixed alcohol with prescription drugs. It is best to work with a professional when you have a problem. Using alcohol doesn't help you feel better when you are depressed, and it may make you feel worse. He made a mistake—a very big mistake. *Impact:* The mother and daughter accept the lack of control inherent in realizing that you cannot stop others from making mistakes, potentially benefit from the a truthful statement about high-risk behavior, and feel some compassion for the victim.

More times than not, survivors have to make difficult decisions about filling in the blanks, and they lack skills for working on this difficult task from the perspective of the present. I often encourage survivors to practice telling their reformed stories as a way of gaining information about the workability of the new story. I also provide skill work to help them deal with difficult words (e.g., *guilt* and *blame*). I start with having the survivor say the words *milk–milk–milk–milk* and notice the associated sensory experiences (e.g., creamy, white, and yummy). Next, I have the survivor continue with *milk–milk–milk–milk* until all of the sensory images vanish. Then I move to words and phrases such as "it's your fault"—"it's your fault"—"it's your fault." I ask the survivors to notice the sensations in their bodies and make room for them. Then we move on to repeating the word or phrase until it is de-literalized. I often explain that the mind is a crown of diamonds (helps us construct more accurate stories that help our lives work) and a crown of thorns (draws us out of the present moment, in which we can make a choice and engage in a new behavior, and into memories and anticipated traumas, in which we often repeat behavior that limits vitality in life).

Survivors need to learn to see the self as a context rather than content during this stage of treatment. To facilitate this process experientially, I typically use two exercises, both of which are ACT strategies. The first is a chessboard metaphor. I ask the survivors to take one position on an issue in the story (it was a choice the suicide victim made) and to watch what the mind offers up in response (it was not a choice the victim made). We then talk about the way mental activity is organized (e.g., is/is not, yes/but, this/not that) and practice visualizing thoughts as chess pieces in a game of chess being played on a board of vast expanse. I encourage survivors to think of self as the chessboard, rather than a knight or queen. As homework, I often suggest that the survivors practice moving from piece level to board level in their daily lives.

The second exercise for helping survivors develop self as context is the passengers on the bus metaphor. I ask survivors to imagine how their lives can change with the revised story in place and then to imagine getting started in making these changes as if they were bus drivers driving a bus in the direction of a planned location. Then I take out a tablet and ask the survivor to tell me what the mind offers up as obstacles (e.g., you can't do that; people will think you're stupid; no one is going to believe you; they all really think it was your fault; you should be ashamed of yourself—thinking you can go back to school or be in a close relationship). I write down the answers and give them to the survivor, asking that the survivor think of the obstacles as passengers on the bus and encouraging the survivor to keep driving the bus in the planned direction. In a group format, I often have each survivor play the role of the driver while other group members play the roles of passengers and speak of the psychological obstacles from scripts provided by the survivor in the driver's seat. The survivor then has a chance to experiment with alternative ways of responding to internal obstacles to behavior change—arguing with them, ignoring them, or simply noticing them. Invariably, the driving survivors' experience is that they are the best drivers when they simply notice the passengers.

Stage 3: Applying the New Story to the World

In the final phase of treatment, the focus is on clarifying values, identifying personal strengths, and developing committed behavior change plans. Use of the Living Your Values exercise (Figure 11–1) can help the survivor begin to assess and monitor consistency between daily choices and behaviors and valued directions for living that work with the new story about the loss. In this stage, the survivor needs to learn the difference between values and goals. In ACT, values are "verbally construed global desired life consequences" (Hayes et al. 1999, p. 206). Values differ from goals in several important ways. They are more abstract and global and hence can bind verbal goals together. Unlike goals, values are never attained, so they have the ability to direct behavior over longer periods. Discussing values before the start of treatment is a motivation tool. Discussing them early in treatment is a way to reawaken dreams of a once-intended life. Discussion of values in the final stage provides survivors with a context for the many failure experiences they may have encountered in working toward goals and increased resiliency for persevering to increase consistency between values and daily activities through action plans.

The survivor's new story implies valued directions, identifies survivor gifts, and suggests committed behavioral action plans. For example, Mrs. G's new story about her son involved not knowing why her son committed suicide. She became free to be with her grandchildren and not know a specific reason. She could feel all the feelings attenuating loss honestly and openly with her daughter-in-law and grandchildren, and she could feel the joy of being with ones she loved. Mrs. G's committed action plan involved using her gift of enthusiasm for learning to study suicide survivors and to create a survivor Web page for display of resources and brief informational summaries about ways to recover from a loss to suicide. Mr. G's revised story included knowing that he had taught his son about life as best he could. Mr. G's committed action plan concerned using his gift of feeling deeply for others to be a mentor to young adults in his community.

Metaphors in the final stage of treatment include the path up a mountain and riding a bike. I use the path up a mountain metaphor to help survivors understand the difference between values and goals and the importance of cultivating the ability to take an eagle's eye point of view. Living in ways consistent with valued directions is like climbing a mountain. At times, the slope is so steep that one is actually going downhill in pursuit of going to the top. If one is looking only at the path, one does not see progress. If one cultivates the ability to view progress from another mountain, then one can more easily see the switchbacks needed to continue to make progress. I use the riding a bike metaphor to help survivors become sensitive to lapses in progress toward a committed action plan and to self-correct before falling off the bike. Much like a tennis player who takes 14 steps to get in place to hit one ball, it is the 100 small centering moves rather than one giant centering effort that keeps one on the bicycle.

Group Treatment of Survivors of Suicide

Groups offer many advantages for treating survivors of suicide. First, survivors often feel less stigmatized when the stated purpose of care is to help them recover from an experience that happened to them, rather than from a mental disorder. Second, survivors tend to feel they are among a group of individuals who understand their predicament to a great extent. Third, survivors benefit from hearing others work to reform their stories and to get their lives back on track. Fourth, survivors as a group are hardworking and capable of offering a great deal of compassion to one another. Fifth, there are so many survivors in larger communities that groups represent a cost-effective method of providing care that is affordable and accessible to all members of a society.

Issues concerning group treatment include the method of selecting survivors for participation, the selection of leaders, the format, the length and duration of treatment, and the evaluation of outcome. Participants may be self-referred or referred by providers in the community, including primary care providers and behavioral health providers. In most instances, participants are survivors age 18 and older who have lost a loved one to suicide within the past 2–5 years. Leaders may be professionals or community members working in collaboration or under the supervision of professionals. In most cases, community members are themselves survivors and hence have up-front acceptance by group members. In addition, community members often work without reimbursement for their services. The use of community members as group leaders has some disadvantages, however, including the need for time-consuming training and ongoing supervision. Every community setting will have to weigh and evaluate their resources and make a decision about the most viable direction for staffing survivor groups in the community.

Most survivor groups use a semistructured format, and specifics vary from group to group. Table 11–3 presents an outline for an eight-session, 90-

minute group meeting for 8–10 survivors. Each group meeting includes di-
dactic instruction concerning survivor experience and recovery, and several
group members work to tell initial and revised stories about their loss in each
of the eight sessions. As shown in Table 11–3, the final meeting includes the
possibility of planning reunions. Some survivor groups become very cohesive
and plan to continue meeting independently after the formal end of the professionally led group. The group format works well with children, with some
adaptation of the length of group sessions (1 hour rather than 90 minutes)
and the language used in the values work. I also use more artwork projects
(visual and dance) to help children in telling initial and revised stories, and
I involve parents in the last half of the initial, middle, and final meetings. The
specific age range of children in a group can be adjusted to meet the needs of
children waiting to participate to some extent. When numbers allow a more
constricted age range, the following age groupings usually work well: 5–9
years, 10–13 years, and 14–17 years.

Symptom checklists such as the Symptom Checklist–90 (Derogatis et al.
1974) have been used to evaluate adult survivor group participants before and
after participation in the group. This approach allows leaders to evaluate the
overall effectiveness of the group and to identify individual participants who
need follow-up treatment in an individual format. The Pediatric Symptom
Checklist (Jellinek et al. 1988) is a good alternative for children, because it is
a reasonable measure of distress, can be administered in a time-effective manner, and is appropriate for children 4–17 years of age.

Treating Survivors of Suicide in Primary Care Settings

Primary care settings offer many opportunities for identifying and treating
survivors. I encourage behavioral health providers to partner with primary
care providers to support realization of these opportunities. Behavioral health
providers can provide in-service programs for primary care providers and serve
as referral resources for survivors who need more specialized treatment and are
unable or unwilling to access treatment in a group format. Figure 11–2 presents data on health-related quality of life scores for a survivor (Mr. L) I saw
for seven primary care visits over a 16-month period. All visits were less than
30 minutes in duration, so treatment was completed in less than 4 hours.

Table 11–3. Survivors of suicide: a group treatment approach

Session theme	Group and homework activities
1. Getting acquainted, remembering, overview of group	Circle introductions Remembering positive memories, sharing resources The plan of who, what, when, how, why, and therefore (develop schedule of presentations by group members—usually two initial and two revised stories per session for sessions 3–8)
2. Accepting and expressing feelings, minding the mind	Breathing, stretching The who, what, where, when, why—initials
3. Understanding survivor responses, impact of trauma	Remembering our dreams and our loss (*Homework:* create reformed story) Getting needed information The who, what, where, when, why—initials and follow-up
4. Living a vital life now: the directions and the barriers	Share images for all areas of the Living Your Values exercise (*Homework:* identify barriers to moving in valued directions) The who, what, where, when, why—initials and revised
5. Living a vital life now with the barriers as passengers on the bus (metaphor)	Share identified barriers to moving in valued directions Passengers on the bus drama—three or four members The who, what, where, when, why—initials and revised
6. Committed action planning	The who, what, where, when, why—initials and revised Passengers on the bus drama—three or four members In my family, I want to stand for…

Table 11–3.   Survivors of suicide: a group treatment approach *(continued)*

Session theme	Group and homework activities
7. Support systems	The who, what, where, when, why—revised
	Passengers on the bus drama—two or three members
	Who is on my team and what are the gaps?
8. Living the new story	Behavior change plans
	Plan reunions

Mr. L was a middle-aged man who had lost a brother to suicide 12 years before his initial visit. His bereavement had been rekindled by the recent deaths of his father and an uncle. Mr. L had never sought care concerning the loss of his brother to suicide, and most of his concerns in the initial contact concerned loss of the brother and wanting his children to understand the importance of having siblings. Mr. L was succeeding in a job that involved considerable responsibility. Mr. L described his relationship with his wife as good but noted that he and she rarely talked about feelings. When asked, Mr. L voiced concerns about his use of alcohol and cigarettes. Plans developed in the first session included engaging in activities to improve his mood, cultivating more acceptance of his sadness and the ability to cry, practice of a controlled drinking plan, and inquiring about participation in a survivors of suicide group program approximately 25 miles from his home. As shown in Figure 11–2, Mr. L's responses to the Duke Health Profile placed him at the 75th percentile for physical health and at the 50th percentile for mental and social health, the normative group being patients presenting to primary care for treatment.

At the second visit, Mr. L had not made contact with the survivor's group and was reluctant to do so, because it was not convenient and he did not want to participate in a group. Mr. L reported feeling more sad and being more able to let himself cry freely. In addition, he related a great deal of sadness about his oldest daughter's coming graduation from high school. Mr. L had followed through with his behavioral mood improvement plan (was exercising five times per week and going on one outing per week with his wife) and had drunk alcohol on only one occasion. At the third follow-up visit, we talked about Mr. L's brother and the events leading up to the suicide. When we talked about valued directions, Mr. L indicated an interest in returning to school and speaking more honestly with his daughter who was emancipating. All the while, Mr. L continued to experience a great deal of sadness and to allow himself to cry. Mr. L was particularly bereaved during the holiday pe-

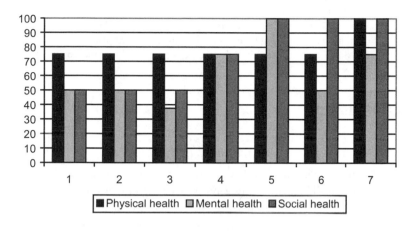

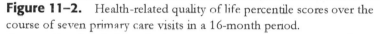

Figure 11–2. Health-related quality of life percentile scores over the course of seven primary care visits in a 16-month period.

Source. Reprinted from Parkerson G: *User's Guide for the Duke Health Profile (DUKE).* Durham, NC, Department of Community and Family Medicine, Duke University Medical Center, 1996. Used with permission.

riod and decided to start taking an antidepressant during a visit with his primary care provider.

In the fourth visit with me, Mr. L related a clear plan for returning to school and active involvement in helping his daughter set up and move into an apartment. He reported having bought himself a pair of tennis shoes for running when he had an unexpected bonus at work. For Mr. L, this recognition of self was a great accomplishment. We focused more specifically on his feelings of guilt and shame about his brother's suicide, and he made a plan to write out his story concerning the brother's death. At the fifth follow-up visit, Mr. L read his story and experienced a great deal of emotion in so doing. He indicated that his brother had responsibility for his choices and that even the most empathetic older brother did not have the power or authority to make choices for a younger brother. Mr. L's fifth-session homework included focusing on reasons he might be angry, because this was the most difficult emotion for him to experience in relation to his brother's suicide. At the sixth follow-up visit, Mr. L further reshaped his story, and his scores in physical and social health were at the one hundredth percentile at the final follow-up visit. Mr. L planned to meet with his physician and make a plan concerning tapering from his antidepressant, because he wanted to experience all of his feelings fully. Mr. L plans one more follow-up visit with me in 2 months to discuss continuation of his committed action plans. He no longer engages in problem use of alcohol; he continues to exercise five times weekly; he is taking pride in his parenting; and he is succeeding in school and plans to graduate within the next 6 months. Mr. L will invite everyone in his family to a graduation party.

Conclusion

We must not turn our back on survivors of suicide. They are our neighbors, our co-workers, and our children's friends. Better identification of children who are survivors is a priority, because they are detected even less often than adult survivors. There are many ways of reaching out to survivors, and all need to be pursued. I am particularly interested in seeing more detection and intervention programs for survivors in primary care settings and schools. We need to continue to evaluate and improve well-established approaches such as survivors of suicide groups and postvention programs. To succeed, we need to follow a theoretical basis for providing care to survivors, and I am recommending the ACT model for this purpose. With a theoretical model such as ACT, we can hope to better understand the processes underlying successful treatment and perhaps do a better job of identifying more vulnerable survivors earlier, so that their suffering has a less deleterious impact on their functioning.

References

Allen BG, Calhoun LG, Cann A, et al: The effect of cause of death on responses to the bereaved: suicide compared to accidental and natural causes. Omega: Journal of Death and Dying 28:39–48, 1993–1994

Brent DA, Peters MJ, Weller E: Resolved: several weeks of depressive symptoms after exposure to a friend's suicide is "major depressive disorder." J Am Acad Child Adolesc Psychiatry 33:582–587, 1994

Calhoun LG, Allen BG: The suicidal death of a child: social perception of stepparents. Omega: Journal of Death and Dying 26:301-307, 1992–1993

Callahan J: Negative effects of a school suicide postvention program: a case example. Crisis 17:108–115, 1996

Derogatis LR, Rickels K, Uhlenhuth EH, et al: The Hopkins Symptom Checklist: a measure of primary symptom dimensions, in Psychological Measurements in Psychopharmacology: Problems in Pharmacopsychiatry. Edited by Pichot P. Basel, Switzerland, Karger, 1974

Elliott DM: Traumatic events: prevalence and delayed recall in the general population. J Consult Clin Psychol 65:811–820, 1997

Farberow NL, Gallagher-Thompson D, Gilewski M, et al: Changes in grief and mental health of bereaved spouses of older suicides. J Gerontol 47:357–366, 1992a

Farberow NL, Gallagher-Thompson D, Gilewski M, et al: The role of social support in the bereavement process of surviving spouses of suicide and natural death. Suicide Life Threat Behav 22:107–124, 1992b

Gaffney DA, Jones ET, Dunne-Maxim K: Support groups for sibling suicide survivors. Crisis 13:76–81, 1992

Grad OT: Similarities and differences in the process of bereavement after suicide and after traffic accidents in Slovenia. Omega: Journal of Death and Dying 33:243–251, 1996a

Grad OT: Suicide: how to survive as a survivor? Crisis 17:136–142, 1996b

Hayes SC, Strosahl KD, Wilson KG: Acceptance and Commitment Therapy: An Experiential Approach to Behavior Change. New York, Guilford, 1999

Jellinek MS, Murphy JM, Robinson J, et al: Pediatric Symptom Checklist: screening school-age children for psychosocial dysfunction. J Pediatr 112:201–209, 1988

Knieper AJ: The suicide survivor's grief and recovery. Suicide Life Threat Behav 29:353–364, 1999

Kroenke K, Spitzer RL, Williams JBW: The PHQ-9: validity of a brief depression severity measure. J Gen Intern Med 16:606–613, 2001

Kubany ES, Haynes SN, Leisen MB, et al: Development and preliminary validation of a brief broad-spectrum measure of trauma exposure: the Traumatic Life Events Questionnaire. Psychol Assess 12:210–224, 2000

Moore MM: Counseling survivors of suicide: implications for group postvention. Journal for Specialists in Group Work 20:40–47, 1995

Orcutt HK: Forgiveness and emotional avoidance: relations with global mental health, physical health, and PTSD symptoms. Poster presented at the 36th annual Association for the Advancement of Behavior Therapy convention, Reno, NV, November 2002

Parkerson G: User's Guide for the Duke Health Profile (DUKE). Durham, NC, Duke University Medical Center, Department of Community and Family Medicine, 1996. Manual available from author at Department of Community and Family Medicine, Box 3886, Duke University Medical Center, Durham, NC 22710.

Pfeffer CR, Martins P, Mann J, et al: Child survivors of suicide: psychosocial characteristics. J Am Acad Child Adolesc Psychiatry 36:65–74, 1997

Reed MD: Sudden death and bereavement outcomes: the impact of resources on grief
symptomatology and detachment. Suicide Life Threat Behav 23:204–220, 1993

Reed MD, Greenwald JY: Survivor-victim status, attachment, and sudden death bereavement. Suicide Life Threat Behav 21:385–401, 1991

Robinson P: Living Life Well: New Strategies for Hard Times. Reno, NV, Context
Press, 1996

Saarinen P, Viinamäki H, Hintikka J, et al: Psychological symptoms of close relatives
of suicide victims. Eur J Psychiatry 13:33–39, 1999

Seguin M, Lesage A, Kiely MC: Parental bereavement after suicide and accident: a
comparative study. Suicide Life Threat Behav 25:489–498, 1995b

Silverman E: Bereavement from suicide as compared to other forms of bereavement.
Omega: Journal of Death and Dying 30:41–51, 1994–1995

Stroebe M, Stroebe W, Schut H, et al: Does disclosure of emotions facilitate recovery
from bereavement: evidence from two prospective studies. J Consult Clin Psychol
70:169–178, 2002

Strosahl K: Building integrated primary care behavioral health delivery systems that
work: a compass and a horizon, in Behavioral Health in Primary Care: A Guide
for Clinical Integration. Edited by Cummings N, Johnson JJ. Madison, CT, Psychosocial Press, 1997, pp 37–58

Wagner KG, Calhoun LG: Perceptions of social support by suicide survivors and their
social networks. School Psychology International 12(1–2):17–23, 1991–1992

Williams JMG: Mindfulness-based cognitive therapy for depression: a new approach
to preventing relapse. Workshop presentation at the ACT, RFT & the New Behavioral Psychology First World Conference, Linkoping, Sweden, August 13–17,
2003

Selected Readings

Grad OT: Suicide of a patient: gender differences in bereavement reactions of therapists.
Suicide Life Threat Behav 27:379–386, 1997

Robinson P: Behavioral health services in primary care: a new perspective for treating
depression. Clin Psychol 5:77–93, 1998

Robinson P: Treating depression in primary care, in Innovations in Clinical Practice:
A Source Book, 1999 Edition. Edited by Vandecreek L, Jackson TL. Sarasota,
FL, Professional Resource Press, 1999

Robinson P: Cost offset opportunities in primary care treatment of depression, in Integrated Behavioral Health Treatments. Edited by Hayes S, Fischer J, O'Donohoe W. Reno, NV, University of Reno, 2002, pp 145–165

Robinson P, Strosahl K: Improving outcomes for a primary care population: depression as an example, in Handbook of Psychological Assessment in Primary Care Settings. Edited by Maruis M. Hillsdale, NJ, Lawrence Erlbaum, 2000, pp 687–711

Strosahl K: Confessions of a behavior therapist in primary care: the odyssey and the ecstasy. Cogn Behav Pract 8:1–28, 1997

Appendix A
Philosophies About Suicide

I. Suicide Is Wrong

1. Suicide does violence to the dignity of human life.
2. Suicide is against basic human nature.
3. Suicide is an oversimplified response to a complex and ambivalent situation.
4. Suicide is a crime against the state.
5. Suicide is an irrevocable act that denies future learning or growth.
6. It is only for God to give and to take away human life. Suicide is rebellion against God.
7. Suicide does violence to the natural order of things.
8. Suicide is not different from homicide.
9. Suicide adversely affects the survivors.

II. Suicide Is Sometimes Permissible

Suicide is permissible when in the individual's view of things the alternatives are unbearable. An example is extreme and incurable physical pain.

III. Suicide Is Not a Moral or Ethical Issue

1. Suicide is a phenomenon of life that is subject to study in the same way that any other phenomena of life should be studied.
2. Suicide represents neither a morally good nor a morally bad action and is an action that takes place beyond the realm of reason.
3. Suicide is a morally neutral act in that every person has a free will and has the right to move and act according to that will.

305

IV. Suicide Is a Positive Response to Certain Conditions

1. When life ceases to be enjoyable or pleasurable, one has the right to end his or her life.
2. A person has the innate right to make any decision, provided it is based on rationality and logical thinking. This includes the right to suicide.
3. There are certain times in life when death is less an evil than is dishonor.
4. Some suicides are demanded by society as a way of dispensing justice.
5. Suicide is a permissible act when it is performed for some great purpose that transcends the value of the human life.

V. Suicide Has Intrinsic Positive Value

1. One must affirm one's self and make decisions. Suicide may be an affirmation of a person's soul, in which case it is fulfillment to carry through this action, and it would be morally wrong for anyone to interfere with this decision.
2. Suicide is sometimes a way to save face, as in the case of hara-kiri, after the individual has lost his or her honor.
3. Suicide has positive value when it provides the means by which a person can enter a meaningful afterlife that he or she desires.
4. Suicide is a way to embrace a personified and eroticized death.
5. Suicide has positive value because it is a way in which one can be immediately reunited with valued ancestors and with loved ones.

Appendix B

Consequences of Suicidal Behavior Questionnaire

Sometimes people with problems attempt suicide. On the lines provided below, write all of the things that might happen if, for whatever reason, you were to *attempt suicide but not die as a result* of your attempt. For each item you list, indicate whether you feel that the result is *mostly good* or *mostly bad,* and then indicate how *important* you feel that result is. Try to think of at least four results. However, if you cannot think of that many, just leave one or more lines blank. Do your best.

Result 1: _____

O = Bad O = Good
Not at all important O1 O2 O3 O4 O5 Extremely important

Result 2: _____

O = Bad O = Good
Not at all important O1 O2 O3 O4 O5 Extremely important

Result 3:_____

O = Bad O = Good
Not at all important O1 O2 O3 O4 O5 Extremely important

Result 4:_____

O = Bad O = Good
Not at all important O1 O2 O3 O4 O5 Extremely important

If you were to *commit suicide,* that is, if you were to die as a result of a suicide attempt, what are all the things that would happen as a result?

To you after death:

Result 1:_____

○ = Bad ○ = Good

Not at all important ○1 ○2 ○3 ○4 ○5 Extremely important

Result 2:_____

○ = Bad ○ = Good

Not at all important ○1 ○2 ○3 ○4 ○5 Extremely important

To those left behind:

Result 1:_____

○ = Bad ○ = Good

Not at all important ○1 ○2 ○3 ○4 ○5 Extremely important

Result 2:_____

○ = Bad ○ = Good

Not at all important ○1 ○2 ○3 ○4 ○5 Extremely important

If you were to *commit suicide,* what reasons do you think you would have for doing it?

Reason 1: _____

Reason 2: _____

Reason 3: _____

Reason 4: _____

When other people *attempt suicide but do not die* as a result, why do you think they do it?

Reason 1: _____

Reason 2: _____

Reason 3: _____

Reason 4: _____

When other people *commit suicide,* why do you think they do it?

Reason 1: _____

Reason 2: _____

Reason 3: _____

Reason 4: _____

Appendix C

Reasons for Living Inventory

Survival and Coping Beliefs

1. I care enough about myself to live.
2. I believe I can find other solutions to my problems.
3. I still have many things left to do.
4. I have hope that things will improve and the future will be happier.
5. I have the courage to face life.
6. I want to experience all that life has to offer, and there are many experiences I haven't had yet that I want to have.
7. I believe everything has a way of working out for the best.
8. I believe I can find a purpose in life, a reason to live.
9. I have a love of life.
10. No matter how badly I feel, I know that it will not last.
11. Life is too beautiful and precious to end it.
12. I am happy and content with my life.
13. I am curious about what will happen in the future.
14. I see no reason to hurry death along.
15. I believe I can learn to adjust or cope with my problems.
16. I believe killing myself would not really accomplish or solve anything.
17. I have a desire to live.
18. I am too stable to kill myself.
19. I have plans I am looking forward to carrying out.
20. I do not believe that things get miserable or hopeless enough that I would rather be dead.
21. I do not want to die.
22. Life is all we have and is better than nothing.
23. I believe I have control over my life and destiny.

Responsibility to Family

1. I would hurt my family too much and I would not want them to suffer.
2. I would not want my family to feel guilty afterward.
3. I would not want my family to think I was selfish or a coward.
4. My family depends on me and needs me.
5. I love and enjoy my family too much and could not leave them.
6. My family might believe I did not love them.
7. I have a responsibility and commitment to my family.

Child-Related Concerns

1. The effect on my children could be harmful.
2. It would not be fair to leave the children for others to take care of.
3. I want to watch my children as they grow.

Fear of Suicide

1. I am afraid of the actual "act" of killing myself (the pain, blood, violence).
2. I am a coward and do not have the guts to do it.
3. I am so inept that my method would not work.
4. I am afraid that my method of killing myself would fail.
5. I am afraid of the unknown.
6. I am afraid of death.
7. I could not decide where, when, and how to do it.

Fear of Social Disapproval

1. Other people would think I am weak and selfish.
2. I would not want people to think I did not have control over my life.
3. I am concerned what others would think of me.

Moral Objections

1. My religious beliefs forbid it.
2. I believe only God has the right to end a life.
3. I consider it morally wrong.
4. I am afraid of going to hell.

Appendix D

Suicidal Thinking and Behaviors Questionnaire

1. Since the first time you thought of suicide, how have your suicidal thoughts changed in intensity?

    ○ 1   ○ 2   ○ 3   ○ 4   ○ 5
    decreased   the same   increased

2. Have you thought about killing yourself in the past 24 hours?

    ○ No   ○ Yes

3. When you think of killing yourself, what are the most important problems you are having that cause you to have these thoughts?

4. Before coming to this office, have you ever told someone that you were thinking of committing suicide?

    ○ No   ○ Yes

5. How many times have you attempted suicide, that is, intentionally physically injured yourself in a manner which, at the time, you or someone else considered a suicide attempt? _____

6. Would any of your problems be solved if you killed yourself?

    ○ 1   ○ 2   ○ 3   ○ 4   ○ 5

    Definitely no   Definitely yes

7. How many people love or care for you? _____

8. Among the people who love or care for you, how many are capable of helping you? _____

9. Do you personally know anyone who committed or attempted suicide?

    ○ No   ○ Yes

Appendix E

Malpractice Management Assessment

Instructions: Please review Chapter 2 ("The Clinician's Emotions, Values, Legal Exposure, and Ethics") and then rate how your clinical practice, charting and documentation, and office policies stack up against our recommended strategies.

Recommended practice	Compliance rating 1 = none 3 = somewhat 5 = completely	Actions to be taken to improve compliance rating
Chart note should document specific suicidal assessment data, interpretation, and clinical decision		
Seek thorough informed consent regarding treatment, alternatives, risks, and benefits from patient and (if available) immediate family members		

Recommended practice	Compliance rating 1 = none 3 = somewhat 5 = completely	Actions to be taken to improve compliance rating
With suicidal patient, reassess suicidality at every visit and note in chart, along with alteration (if any) in treatment plan		
Document the findings and recommendations of any team review, peer-to-peer consultation		
Briefly document the evidence base for assessment and treatment methods and settings you elect to use		
Reduce documentation of "canned" suicide prevention tactics as proof of suicidal risk management		
Reduce policy-driven treatment directives for suicidal behavior; emphasize clinical decision making of the provider		

Index

*Page numbers printed in **boldface** type refer to tables or figures.*